The Complete Mediterranean Diet Cookbook

Amazing Healthy Recipes to Discover Mediterranean Diet and Improve Your Lifestyle

I0145891

America Best Recipes

Table of contents

Banana and Quinoa Casserole

Preparation Time: 10 minutes

Cooking Time: 1 hour and 20 minutes

Servings: 8

Ingredients:

- 3 cups bananas, peeled and mashed
- ¼ cup pure maple syrup
- ¼ cup molasses
- 1 tbsp. cinnamon powder
- 2 tsp. vanilla extract
- 1 tsp. cloves, ground
- 1 tsp. ginger, ground
- ½ tsp. allspice, ground
- 1 cup quinoa
- ¼ cup almonds, chopped
- 2 and ½ cups almond milk

Directions:

1. In a baking dish, combine the bananas with the maple syrup, molasses and the rest of the ingredients, toss and bake at 350°F for 1 hour and 20 minutes.
2. Divide the mix between plates and serve for breakfast.

Nutrition: Calories 213, Fat 4.1g, Carbs 41 g, Protein 4.5 g

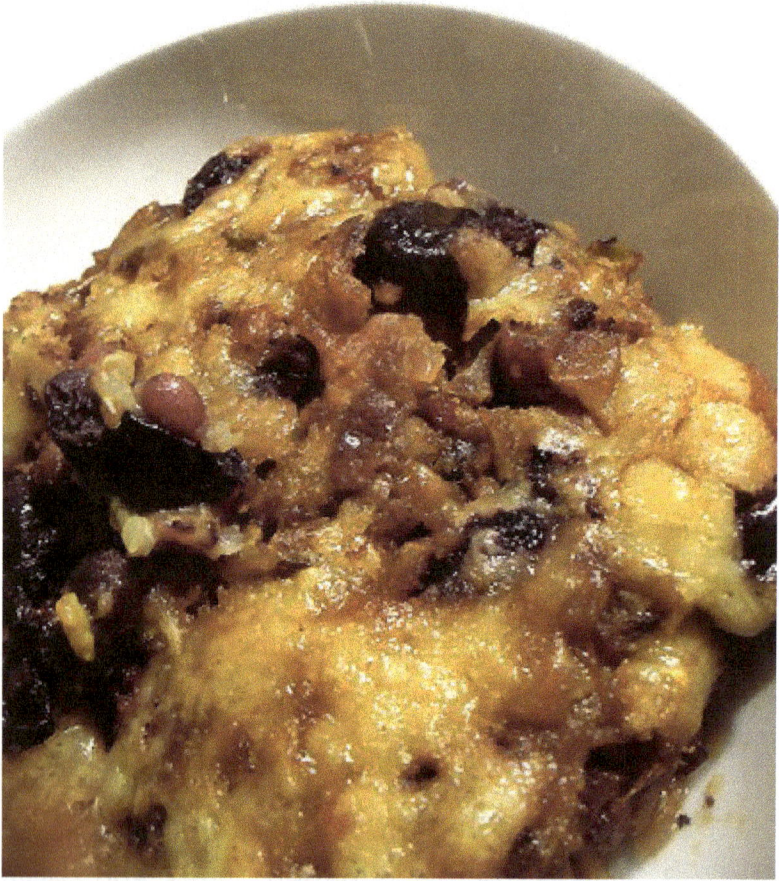

Ham Muffins

Preparation Time: 10 minutes

Cooking Time: 15 minutes

Servings: 6

Ingredients:

- 9 ham slices
- 5 eggs, whisked
- 1/3 cup spinach, chopped
- ¼ cup feta cheese, crumbled
- ½ cup roasted red peppers, chopped
- A pinch of salt and black pepper
- 1 and ½ tbsp. basil pesto
- Cooking spray

Directions:

1. Grease a muffin tin with cooking spray and line each muffin mould with 1 and ½ ham slices.
2. Divide the peppers and the rest of the ingredients except the eggs, pesto, salt and pepper into the ham cups.
3. In a bowl, mix the eggs with the pesto, salt and pepper, whisk and pour over the peppers mix.

4. Bake the muffins in the oven at 400°F for 15 minutes and serve for breakfast.

Nutrition: Calories 109 g, Fat 6.7 g, Carbs 1.8 g, Protein 9.3 g

Cheesy Yogurt

Preparation Time: 4 hours and 5 minutes

Cooking Time: 0 minutes

Servings: 4

Ingredients:

- 1 cup Greek yogurt
- 1 tbsp. honey
- ½ cup feta cheese, crumbled

Directions:

- In a blender, combine the yogurt with the honey and the cheese and pulse well.
- Divide into bowls and freeze for 4 hours before serving for breakfast.

Nutrition: Calories 161, Fat 11.5 g, Carbs 36.6 g, Protein 15.4 g

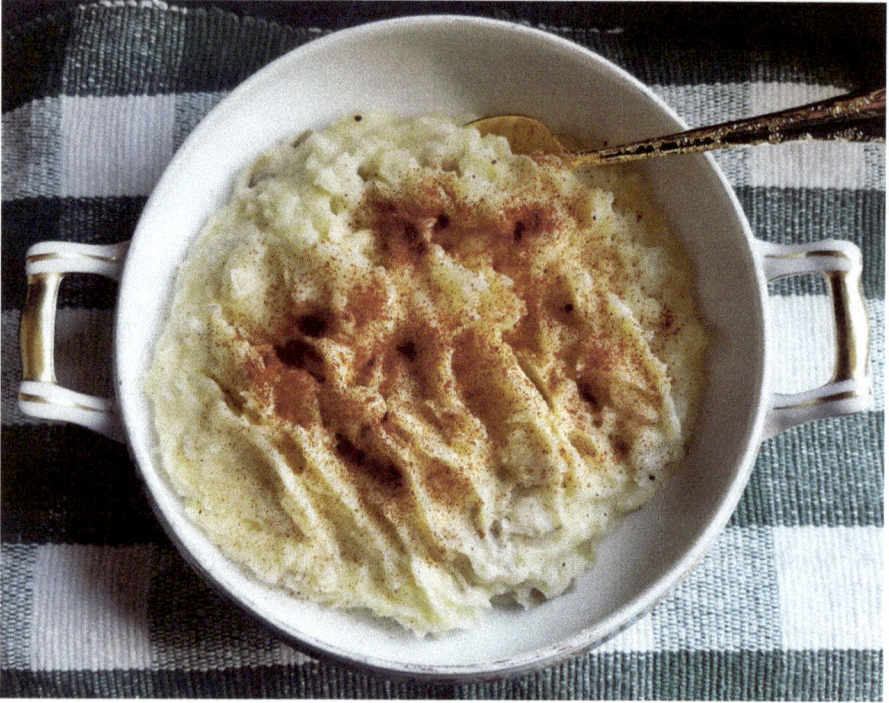

Avocado Spread

Preparation Time: 5 minutes

Cooking Time: 0 minutes

Servings: 8

Ingredients:

- 2 avocados, peeled, pitted and roughly chopped
- 1 tbsp. sun-dried tomatoes, chopped
- 2 tbsp. lemon juice
- 3 tbsp. cherry tomatoes, chopped
- ¼ cup red onion, chopped
- 1 tsp. oregano, dried
- 2 tbsp. parsley, chopped
- 4 kalamata olives, pitted and chopped
- A pinch of salt and black pepper

Directions:

1. Put the avocados in a bowl and mash with a fork.
2. Add the rest of the ingredients, stir to combine and serve as a morning spread.

Nutrition:

Calories 110,

Fat 10.5 g,

Fiber 3.6 g,

Carbs 5.6 g,

Protein 1.4 g

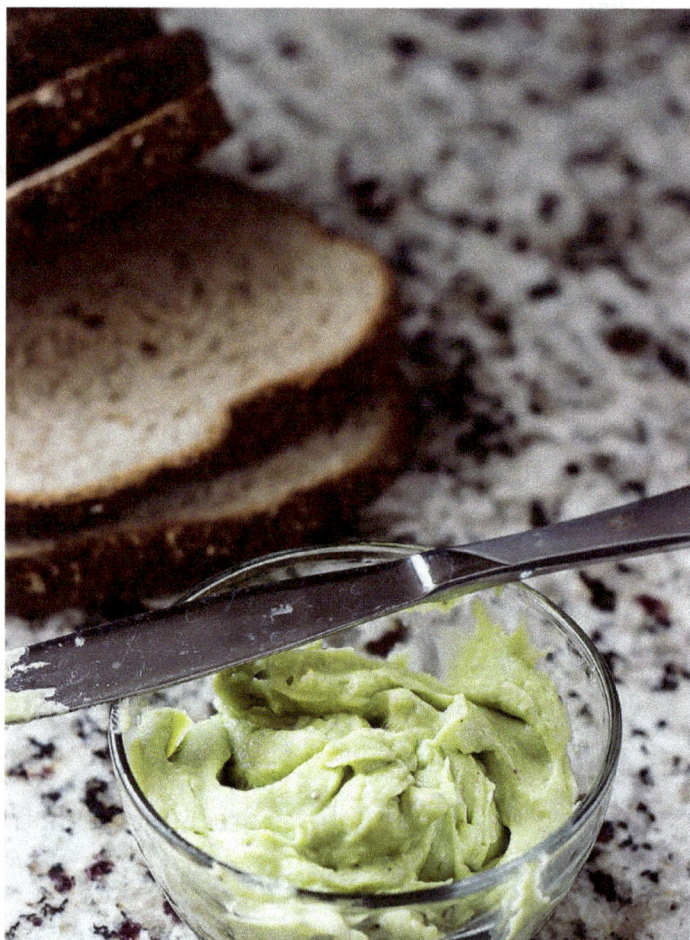

Artichokes and Cheese Omelet

Preparation Time: 10 minutes

Cooking Time: 8 minutes

Servings: 1

Ingredients:

- 1 tsp. avocado oil
- 1 tbsp. almond milk
- 2 eggs, whisked
- A pinch of salt and black pepper
- 2 tbsp. tomato, cubed
- 2 tbsp. kalamata olives, pitted and sliced
- 1 artichoke heart, chopped
- 1 tbsp. tomato sauce
- 1 tbsp. feta cheese, crumbled

Directions:

1. In a bowl, combine the eggs with the milk, salt, pepper and the rest of the ingredients except the avocado oil and whisk well.
2. Heat up a pan with the avocado oil over medium-high heat, add the omelet mix, spread into the pan, cook for 4 minutes, flip, cook for 4 minutes more, transfer to a plate and serve.

Nutrition:

Calories 303,

Fat 17.5 g,

Fiber 9.6 g,

Carbs 6.6 g,

Protein 15.4 g

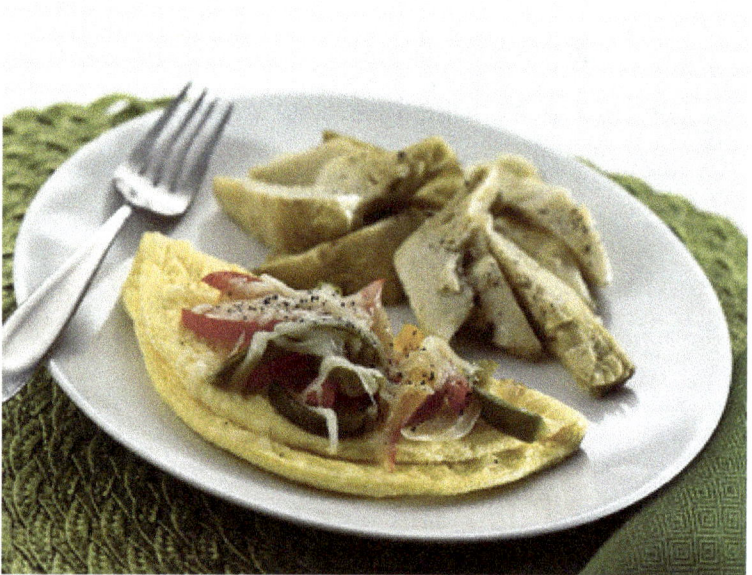

Walnut Poached Eggs

Preparation Time: 10 minutes

Cooking Time: 10 minutes

Servings: 2

Ingredients:

- 2 slices whole grain bread toasted
- 1 oz sun-dried tomato, sliced
- 1 tbsp. cream cheese
- 1/3 tsp. minced garlic
- 2 slices prosciutto
- 2 eggs
- 1 tbsp. walnuts
- ½ cup fresh basil
- 1 oz Parmesan, grated
- 3 tbsp. olive oil
- ¼ tsp. ground black pepper
- 1 cup water, for cooking

Directions:

1. Pour water in the saucepan and bring it to boil.
2. Then crack eggs in the boiling water and cook them for 3-4 minutes or until the egg whites are white.

3.   Meanwhile, churn together minced garlic and cream cheese.

4.   Spread the bread slices with the cream cheese mixture.

5.   Top them with the sun-dried tomatoes.

6.   Make the pesto sauce: Blend together ground black pepper, Parmesan, olive oil, and basil. When the mixture is homogenous, pesto is cooked.

7.   Carefully transfer the poached eggs over the sun-dried tomatoes and sprinkle with pesto sauce.

8.   The poached eggs should be hot while serving.

Nutrition:

Calories 317,

Fat 36.5 g,

Fiber 3.6 g,

Carbs 17.6 g,

Protein 17.4 g

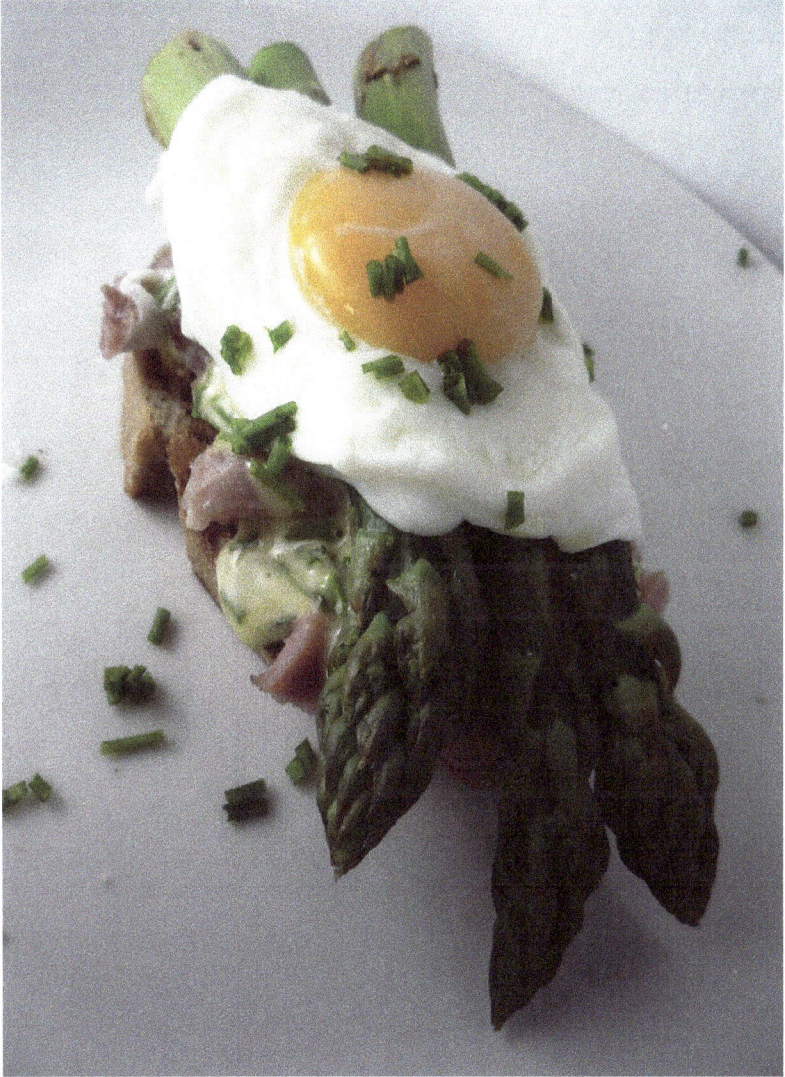

Almond Cream Cheese Bake

Preparation Time: 10 minutes

Cooking Time: 2 hours

Servings: 4

Ingredients:

- 1 cup cream cheese
- 4 tbsp. honey
- 1 oz almonds, chopped
- ½ tsp. vanilla extract
- 3 eggs, beaten
- 1 tbsp. semolina

Directions:

1. Put beaten eggs in the mixing bowl.
2. Add cream cheese, semolina, and vanilla extract.
3. Blend the mixture with the help of the hand mixer until it is fluffy.
4. After this, add chopped almonds and mix up the mass well.
5. Transfer the cream cheese mash in the non-sticky baking mold.
6. Flatten the surface of the cream cheese mash well.
7. Preheat the oven to 325°F.

8. Cook the breakfast for 2 hours.

9. The meal is cooked when the surface of the mash is light brown.

10. Chill the cream cheese mash little and sprinkle with honey.

Nutrition:

Calories 352,

Fat 22.5 g,

Fiber 1.6 g,

Carbs 7.6 g,

Protein 10.4 g

Chili Egg Cups

Preparation Time: 15 minutes

Cooking Time: 15 minutes

Servings: 4

Ingredients:

- 1 tsp. chives, chopped
- 4 eggs
- 1 tsp. tomato paste
- 1 tbsp. Plain yogurt
- ½ tsp. butter, softened
- ¼ tsp. chili flakes
- ½ oz Cheddar cheese, shredded

Directions:

1. Preheat the oven to 365°F.
2. Brush the muffin molds with the softened butter from inside.
3. Then mix up together Plain yogurt with chili flakes and tomato paste.
4. Crack the eggs in the muffin molds.
5. After this, carefully place the tomato paste mixture over the eggs and top with Cheddar cheese.
6. Sprinkle the eggs with chili flakes and place in the preheated oven.

7. Cook the egg cups for 15 minutes.

8. Then check if the eggs are solid and remove them from the oven.

9. Chill the egg cups till the room temperature and gently remove from the muffin molds.

Nutrition:

Calories 85,

Fat 6.5 g,

Fiber 0.6 g,

Carbs 0.6 g,

Protein 6.4 g

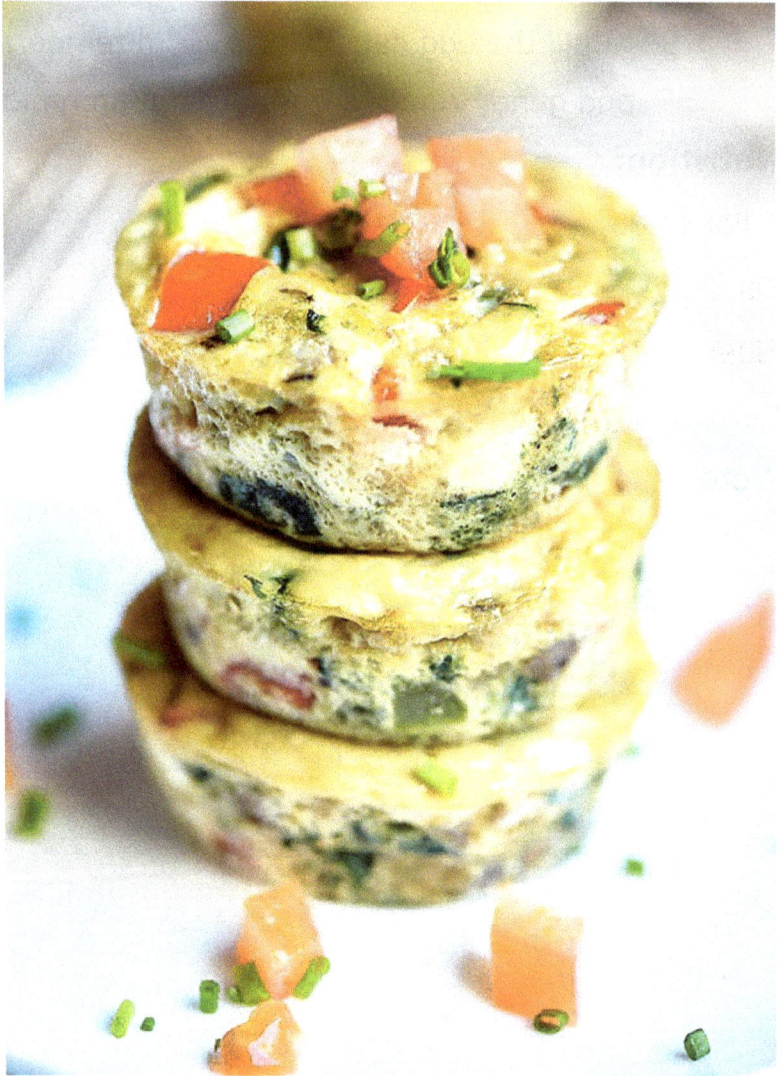

Dill Eggs Mix

Preparation Time: 10 minutes

Cooking Time: 15 minutes

Servings: 2

Ingredients:

- 2 eggs
- 2 oz Feta cheese
- 1 tsp. fresh dill, chopped
- 1 tsp. butter
- ½ tsp. olive oil
- ¼ tsp. onion powder
- ¼ tsp. chili flakes

Directions:

1. Toss butter in the skillet.
2. Add olive oil and bring to boil.
3. After this, crack the eggs in the skillet.
4. Sprinkle them with chili flakes and onion powder.
5. Then preheat the oven to 360°F.
6. Transfer the skillet with eggs in the oven and cook for 10 minutes.
7. Then crumble Feta cheese and sprinkle it over the eggs.
8. Bake the eggs for 5 minutes more.

Nutrition:

Calories 185,

Fat 13.5 g,

Fiber 0.6 g,

Carbs 2.6 g,

Protein 15.4 g

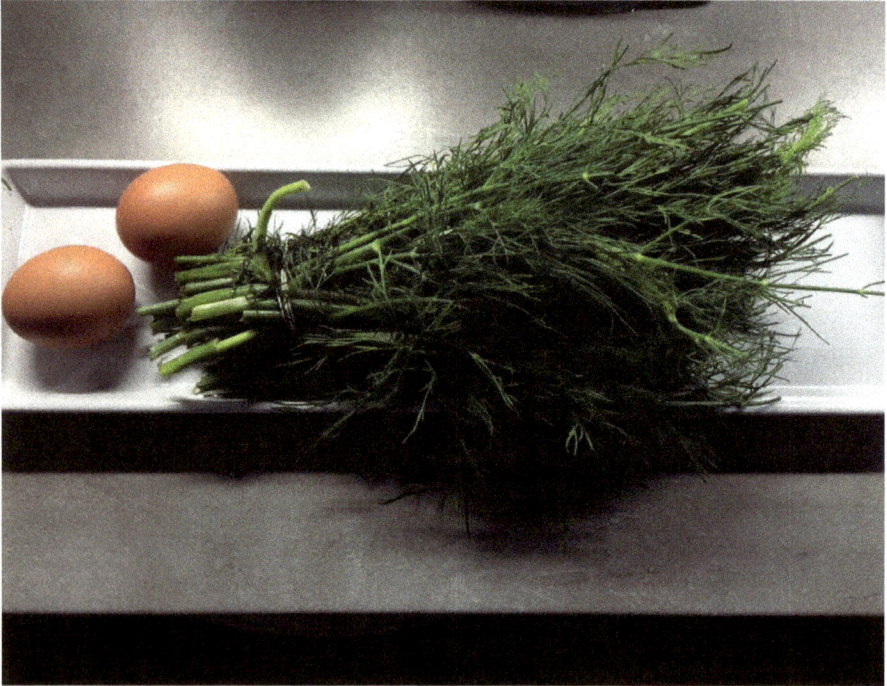

Hummus and Tomato Sandwich

Preparation Time: 10 minutes

Cooking Time: 2 minutes

Servings: 3

Ingredients:

- 6 whole grain bread slices
- 1 tomato
- 3 Cheddar cheese slices
- ½ tsp. dried oregano
- 1 tsp. green chili paste
- ½ red onion, sliced
- 1 tsp. lemon juice
- 1 tbsp. hummus
- 3 lettuce leaves

Directions:

1. Slice tomato into 6 slices.
2. In the shallow bowl mix up together dried oregano, green chili paste, lemon juice, and hummus.
3. Spread 3 bread slices with the chili paste mixture.
4. After this, place the sliced tomatoes on them.

5. Add sliced onion, Cheddar cheese, and lettuce leaves.

6. Cover the lettuce leaves with the remaining bread slices to get the sandwiches.

7. Preheat the grill to 365°F.

8. Grill the sandwiches for 2 minutes.

Nutrition:

Calories 269,

Fat 12.5 g,

Fiber 9.6 g,

Carbs 25.6 g,

Protein 13.4 g

Buttery Pancakes

Preparation Time: 10 minutes

Cooking Time: 10 minutes

Servings: 5

Ingredients:

- 1 cup wheat flour, whole-grain
- 1 tsp. baking powder
- 1 tsp. lemon juice
- 3 eggs, beaten
- ¼ cup Splenda
- 1 tsp. vanilla extract
- 1/3 cup blueberries
- 1 tbsp. olive oil
- 1 tsp. butter
- 1/3 cup milk

Directions:

1. In the mixer bowl, combine together baking powder, wheat flour, lemon juice, eggs, Splenda, vanilla extract, milk, and olive oil.
2. Blend the liquid until it is smooth and homogenous.
3. After this, toss the butter in the skillet and melt it.

4. With the help of the ladle pour the pancake batter in the hot skillet and flatten it in the shape of the pancake.

5. Sprinkle the pancake with the blueberries gently and cook for 1.5 minutes over the medium heat.

6. Then flip the pancake onto another side and cook it for 30 seconds more.

7. Repeat the same steps with all remaining batter and blueberries.

8. Transfer the cooked pancakes in the serving plate.

Nutrition:

Calories 152,

Fat 7.5 g,

Fiber 3.6 g,

Carbs 30.6 g,

Protein 7.4 g

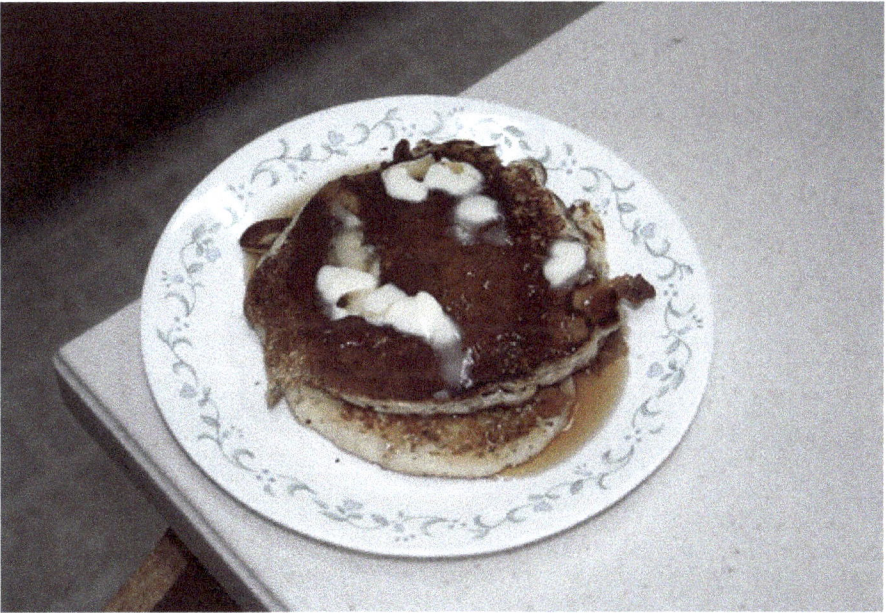

Cream Olive Muffins

Preparation Time: 15 minutes

Cooking Time: 20 minutes

Servings: 6

Ingredients:

- ½ cup quinoa, cooked
- 2 oz Feta cheese, crumbled
- 2 eggs, beaten
- 3 kalamata olives, chopped
- ¾ cup heavy cream
- 1 tomato, chopped
- 1 tsp. butter, softened
- 1 tbsp. wheat flour, whole grain
- ½ tsp. salt

Directions:

1. In the mixing bowl whisk eggs and add Feta cheese.
2. Then add chopped tomato and heavy cream.
3. After this, add wheat flour, salt, and quinoa.
4. Then add kalamata olives and mix up the ingredients with the help of the spoon.
5. Brush the muffin molds with the butter from inside.

6. Transfer quinoa mixture in the muffin molds and flatten it with the help of the spatula or spoon if needed.

7. Cook the muffins in the preheated to 355°F oven for 20 minutes.

Nutrition:

Calories 165,

Fat 10.5 g,

Fiber 1.6 g,

Carbs 11.6 g,

Protein 5.4 g

Herbed Fried Eggs

Preparation Time: 6 minutes

Cooking Time: 7 minutes

Servings: 2

Ingredients:

- 4 eggs
- 1 tbsp. butter
- ½ tsp. chives, chopped
- ½ tsp. fresh parsley, chopped
- 1/3 tsp. fresh dill, chopped
- ¾ tsp. sea salt

Directions:

1. Toss butter in the skillet and bring it to boil.
2. Then crack the eggs in the coiled butter and sprinkle with sea salt.
3. Cook the eggs with the closed lid for 2 minutes over the medium heat.
4. Then open the lid and sprinkle them with parsley, dill, and chives.
5. Cook the eggs for 3 minutes more over the medium heat.
6. Carefully transfer the cooked meal in the plate. Use the wooden spatula for this step.

Nutrition:

Calories 177,

Fat 14.5 g,

Fiber 0.6 g,

Carbs 0.6 g,

Protein 11.4 g

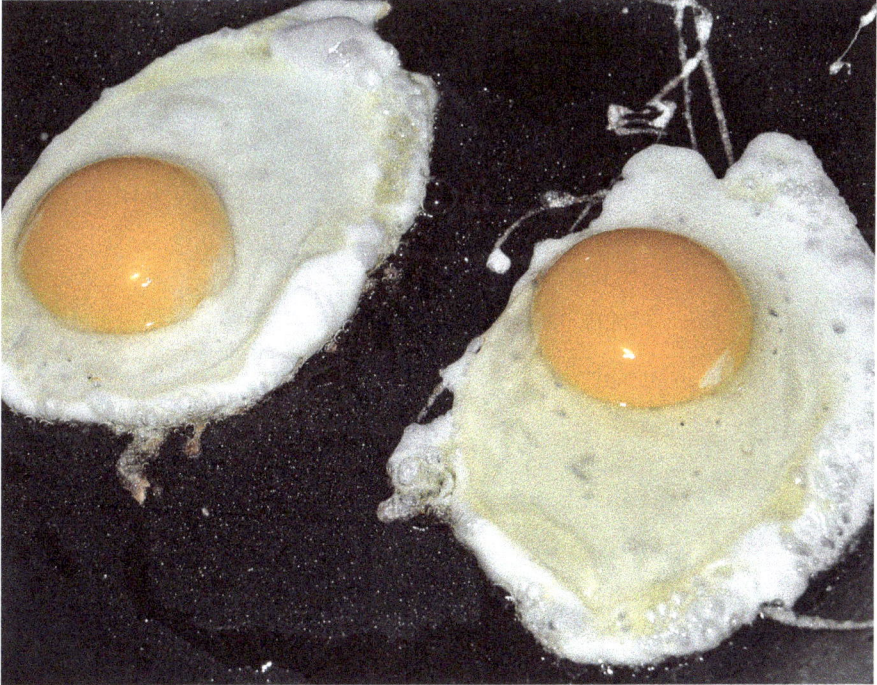

Chili Scramble

Preparation Time: 15 minutes

Cooking Time: 15 minutes

Servings: 4

Ingredients:

- 3 tomatoes
- 4 eggs
- ¼ tsp. of sea salt
- ½ chili pepper, chopped
- 1 tbsp. butter
- 1 cup water, for cooking

Directions:

1. Pour water in the saucepan and bring it to boil.
2. Then remove water from the heat and add tomatoes.
3. Let the tomatoes stay in the hot water for 2-3 minutes.
4. After this, remove the tomatoes from water and peel them.
5. Place butter in the pan and melt it.
6. Add chopped chili pepper and fry it for 3 minutes over the medium heat.

7. Then chop the peeled tomatoes and add into the chili peppers.

8. Cook the vegetables for 5 minutes over the medium heat. Stir them from time to time.

9. After this, add sea salt and crack the eggs

10. Stir (scramble) the eggs well with the help of the fork and cook them for 3 minutes over the medium heat.

Nutrition:

Calories 177,

Fat 7.5 g,

Fiber 1.6 g,

Carbs 4.6 g,

Protein 6.4 g

Couscous and Chickpeas Bowls

Preparation Time: 10 minutes

Cooking Time: 6 minutes

Servings: 4

Ingredients:

- ¾ cup whole wheat couscous
- 1 yellow onion, chopped
- 1 tbsp. olive oil
- 1 cup water
- 2 garlic cloves, minced
- 15 oz. canned chickpeas, drained and rinsed
- A pinch of salt and black pepper
- 15 oz. canned tomatoes, chopped
- 14 oz. canned artichokes, drained and chopped
- ½ cup Greek olives, pitted and chopped
- ½ tsp. oregano, dried
- 1 tbsp. lemon juice

Directions:

1. Put the water in a pot, bring to a boil over medium heat, add the couscous, stir, take off the heat, cover the pan, leave aside for 10 minutes and fluff with a fork.

2. Heat up a pan with the oil over medium-high heat, add the onion and sauté for 2 minutes.

3. Add the rest of the ingredients, toss and cook for 4 minutes more.

4. Add the couscous, toss, divide into bowls and serve for breakfast.

Nutrition:

Calories 540,

Fat 10.5 g,

Fiber 9.6 g,

Carbs 51.6 g,

Protein 11.4 g

Banana Oats

Preparation Time: 10 minutes

Cooking Time: 0 minutes

Servings: 2

Ingredients:

- 1 banana, peeled and sliced
- 1¾ cup almond milk
- ½ cup cold brewed coffee
- 2 dates, pitted
- 2 tbsp. cocoa powder
- 1 cup rolled oats
- 1 and ½ tbsp. chia seeds

Directions:

1. In a blender, combine the banana with the milk and the rest of the ingredients, pulse, divide into bowls and serve for breakfast.

Nutrition:

Calories 451

Fat 25.1 g,

Fiber 9.9 g,

Carbs 55.4 g,

Protein 9.3 g

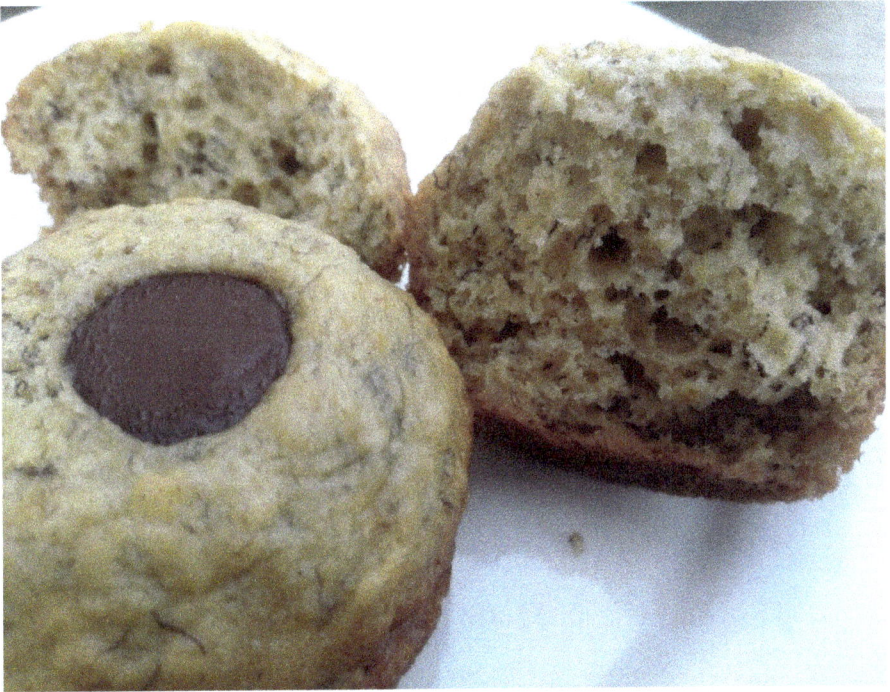

Slow-cooked Peppers Frittata

Preparation Time: 10 minutes

Cooking Time: 3 hours

Servings: 6

Ingredients:

- ½ cup almond milk
- 8 eggs, whisked
- Salt and black pepper to the taste
- 1 tsp. oregano, dried
- 1 and ½ cups roasted peppers, chopped
- ½ cup red onion, chopped
- 4 cups baby arugula
- 1 cup goat cheese, crumbled
- Cooking spray

Directions:

1. In a bowl, combine the eggs with salt, pepper and the oregano and whisk.
2. Grease your slow cooker with the cooking spray, arrange the peppers and the remaining ingredients inside and pour the eggs mixture over them.
3. Put the lid on and cook on Low for 3 hours.
4. Divide the frittata between plates and serve.

Nutrition:

Calories 259,

Fat 20.2,

Fiber 1,

Carbs 4.4,

Protein 16.3

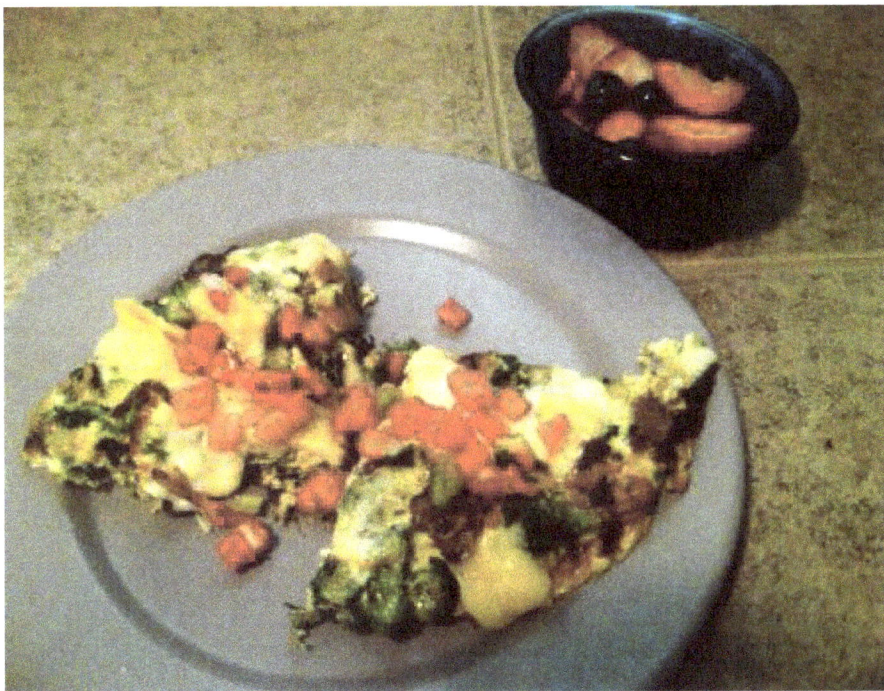

Veggie Bowls

Preparation Time: 10 minutes

Cooking Time: 5 minutes

Servings: 4

Ingredients:

- 1 tbsp. olive oil
- 1 lb. asparagus, trimmed and roughly chopped
- 3 cups kale, shredded
- 3 cups Brussels sprouts, shredded
- ½ cup hummus
- 1 avocado, peeled, pitted and sliced
- 4 eggs, soft boiled, peeled and sliced

For the dressing:

- 2 tbsp. lemon juice
- 1 garlic clove, minced
- 2 tsp. Dijon mustard
- 2 tbsp. olive oil
- Salt and black pepper to the taste

Directions:

1. Heat up a pan with 2 tbsp. oil over medium-high heat, add the asparagus and sauté for 5 minutes stirring often.

2. In a bowl, combine the other 2 tbsp. oil with the lemon juice, garlic, mustard, salt and pepper and whisk well.
3. In a salad bowl, combine the asparagus with the kale, sprouts, hummus, avocado and the eggs and toss gently.
4. Add the dressing, toss and serve for breakfast.

Nutrition:

Calories 323,

Fat 21 g,

Fiber 10.9 g,

Carbs 24.8 g

Avocado and Apple Smoothie

Preparation Time: 5 minutes

Cooking Time: 0 minutes

Servings: 2

Ingredients:

- 3 cups spinach
- 1 green apple, cored and chopped
- 1 avocado, peeled, pitted and chopped
- 3 tbsp. chia seeds
- 1 tsp. honey
- 1 banana, frozen and peeled
- 2 cups coconut water

Directions:

1. In your blender, combine the spinach with the apple and the rest of the ingredients, pulse, divide into glasses and serve.

Nutrition:

Calories 168,

Fat 10.1 g,

Fiber 6 g,

Carbs 21 g,

Protein 2.1 g

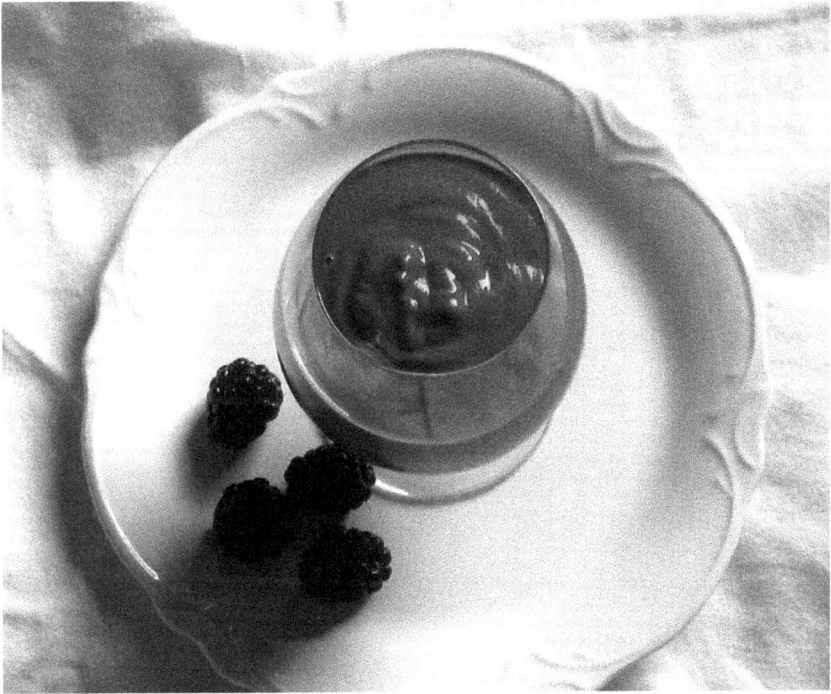

Avocado Toast

Preparation Time: 10 minutes

Cooking Time: 0 minutes

Servings: 2

Ingredients:

- 1 tbsp. goat cheese, crumbled
- 1 avocado, peeled, pitted and mashed
- A pinch of salt and black pepper
- 2 whole wheat bread slices, toasted
- ½ tsp. lime juice
- 1 persimmon, thinly sliced
- 1 fennel bulb, thinly sliced
- 2 tsp. honey
- 2 tbsp. pomegranate seeds

Directions:

1. In a bowl, combine the avocado flesh with salt, pepper, lime juice and the cheese and whisk.
2. Spread this onto toasted bread slices, top each slice with the remaining ingredients and serve for breakfast.

Nutrition:

Calories 348,

Fat 20.8 g

Fiber 12.3 g,

Carbs 38.7 g,

Protein 7.1 g

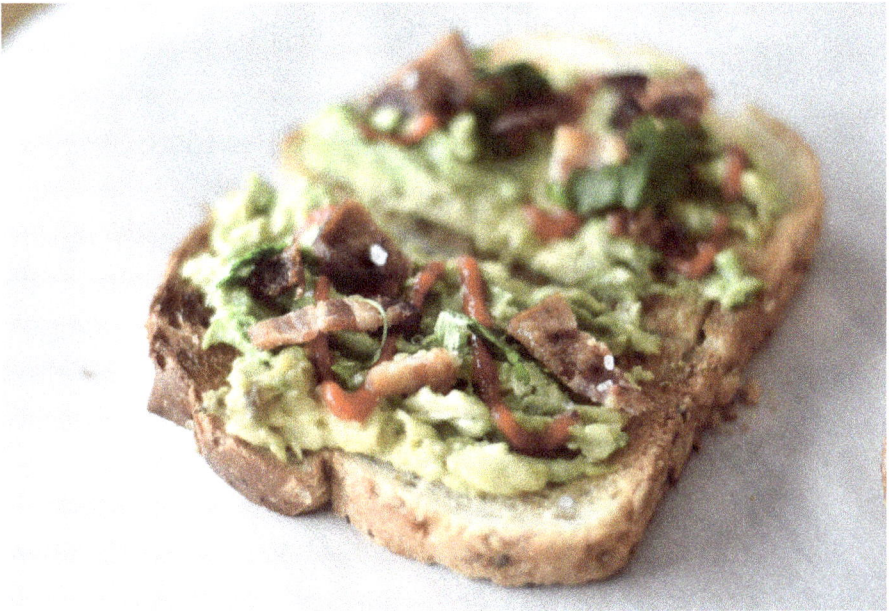

Mini Frittatas

Preparation Time: 5 minutes

Cooking Time: 15 minutes

Servings: 12

Ingredients:

- 1 yellow onion, chopped
- 1 cup parmesan, grated
- 1 yellow bell pepper, chopped
- 1 red bell pepper, chopped
- 1 zucchini, chopped
- Salt and black pepper to the taste
- 8 eggs, whisked
- A drizzle of olive oil
- 2 tbsp. chives, chopped

Directions:

1. Heat up a pan with the oil over medium-high heat, add the onion, the zucchini and the rest of the ingredients except the eggs and chives and sauté for 5 minutes stirring often.
2. Divide this mix on the bottom of a muffin pan, pour the eggs mixture on top, sprinkle salt, pepper and the chives and bake at 350°F for 10 minutes.

3. Serve the mini frittatas for breakfast right away.

Nutrition:

Calories 55,

Fat 3 g,

Fiber 0.7 g,

Carbs 3.2 g,

Protein 4.2 g

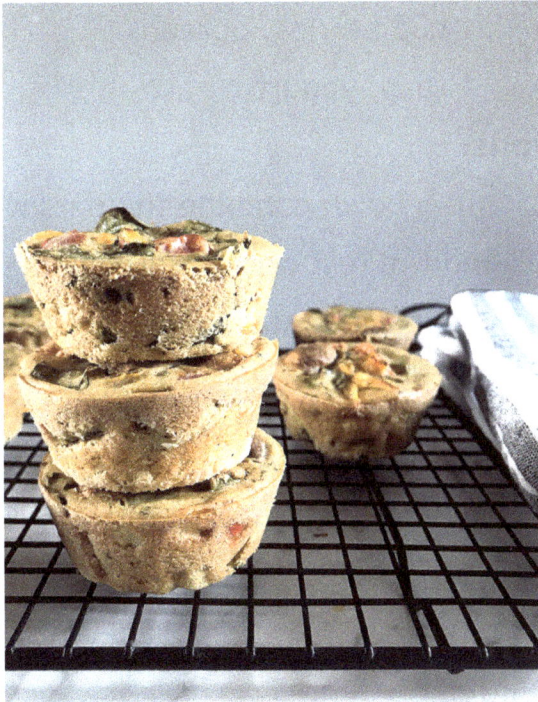

Berry Oats

Preparation Time: 5 minutes

Cooking Time: 0 minutes

Servings: 2

Ingredients :

- ½ cup rolled oats
- 1 cup almond milk
- ¼ cup chia seeds
- A pinch of cinnamon powder
- 2 tsp. honey
- 1 cup berries, pureed
- 1 tbsp. yogurt

Directions:

1. In a bowl, combine the oats with the milk and the rest of the ingredients except the yogurt, toss, divide into bowls, top with the yogurt and serve cold for breakfast.

Nutrition:

Calories 420,

Fat 30.3 g,

Fiber 7.2 g,

Carbs 35.3 g,

Protein 6.4 g

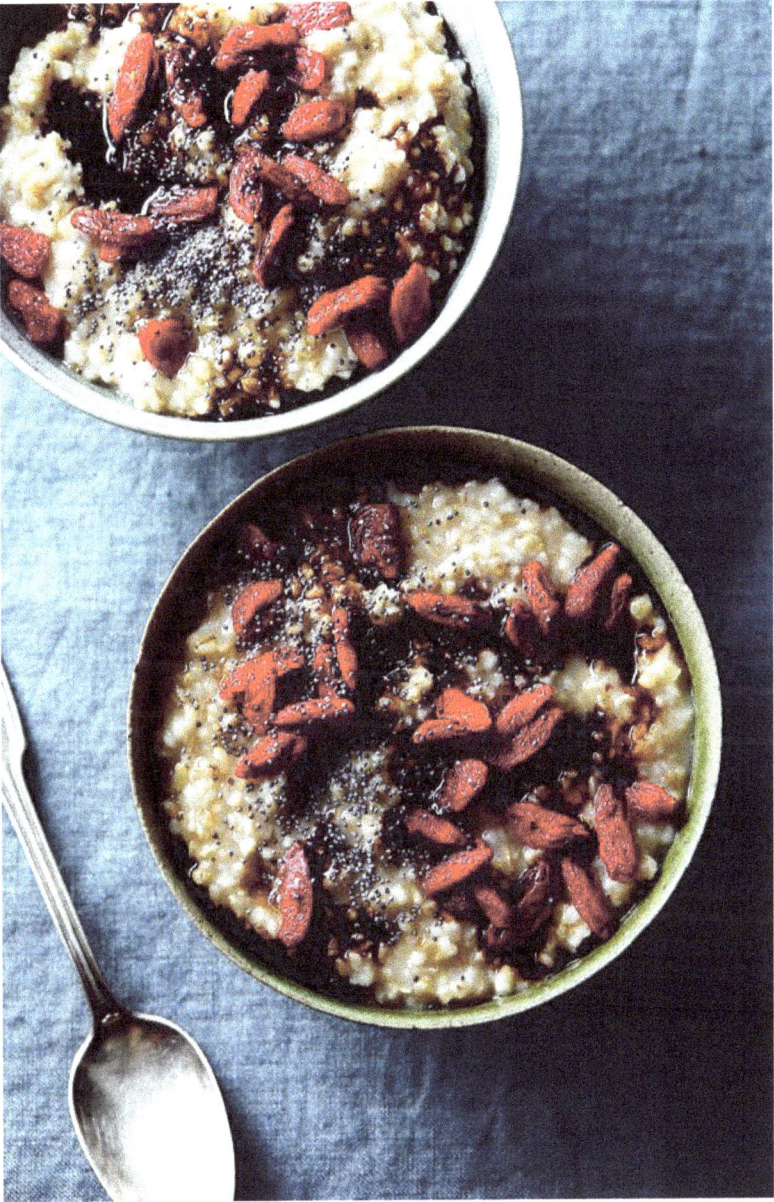

Sun-dried Tomatoes Oatmeal

Preparation Time: 10 minutes

Cooking Time: 25 minutes

Servings: 4

Ingredients:

- 3 cups water
- 1 cup almond milk
- 1 tbsp. olive oil
- 1 cup steel-cut oats
- ¼ cup sun-dried tomatoes, chopped
- A pinch of red pepper flakes

Directions:

1. In a pan, mix the water with the milk, bring to a boil over medium heat.
2. Meanwhile, heat up a pan with the oil over medium-high heat, add the oats, cook them for about 2 minutes and transfer m to the pan with the milk.
3. Stir the oats, add the tomatoes and simmer over medium heat for 23 minutes.
4. Divide the mix into bowls, sprinkle the red pepper flakes on top and serve for breakfast.

Nutrition:

Calories 170,

Fat 17.8 g,

Fiber 1.5 g,

Carbs 3.8 g,

Protein 1.5 g

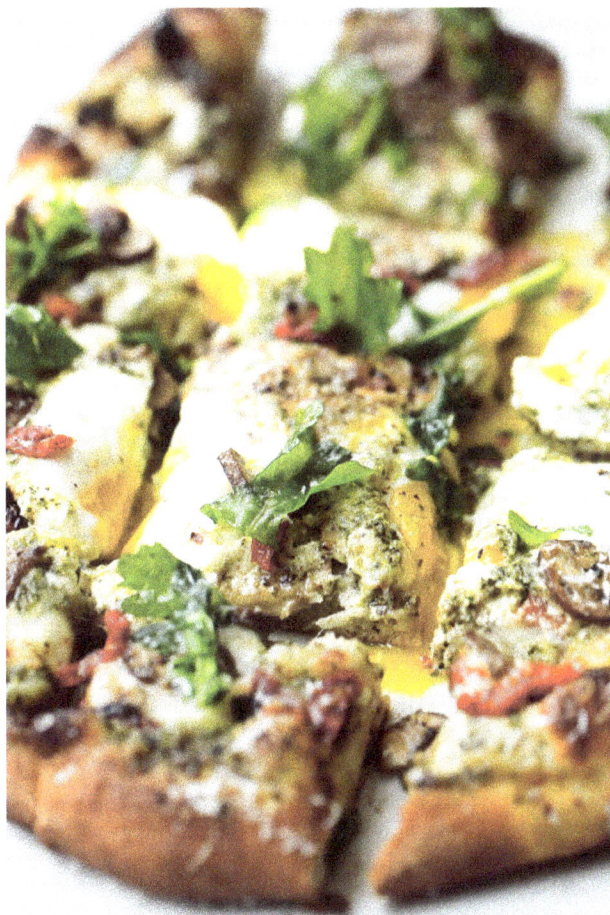

Quinoa Muffins

Preparation Time: 10 minutes

Cooking Time: 30 minutes

Servings: 12

Ingredients:

- 1 cup quinoa, cooked
- 6 eggs, whisked
- Salt and black pepper to the taste
- 1 cup Swiss cheese, grated
- 1 small yellow onion, chopped
- 1 cup white mushrooms, sliced
- ½ cup sun-dried tomatoes, chopped

Directions:

1. In a bowl, combine the eggs with salt, pepper and the rest of the ingredients and whisk well.
2. Divide this into a silicone muffin pan, bake at 350°F for 30 minutes and serve for breakfast.

Nutrition:

Calories 123,

Fat 5.6g,

Fiber 1.3 g,

Carbs 10.8 g,

Protein 7.5 g

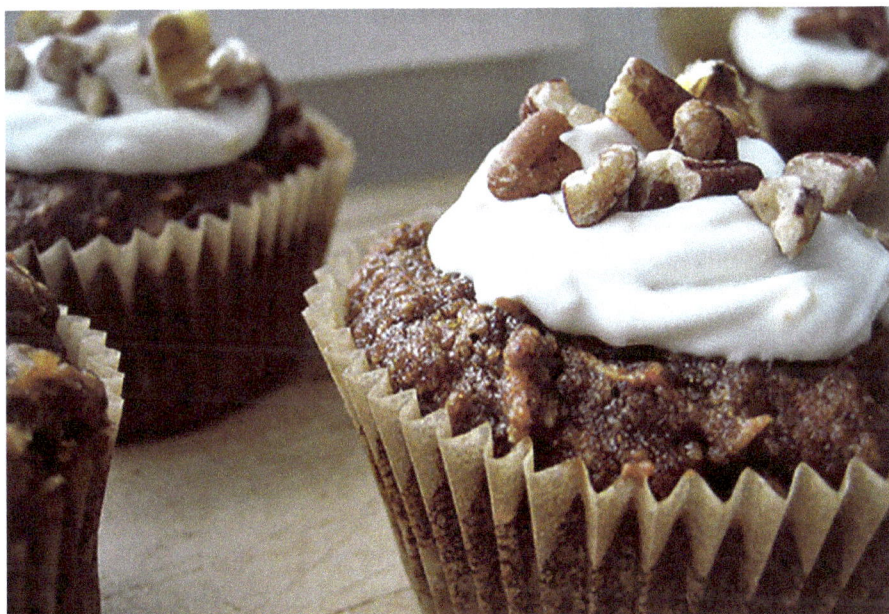

Quinoa and Eggs Pan

Preparation Time: 10 minutes

Cooking Time: 23 minutes

Servings: 4

Ingredients:

- 4 bacon slices, cooked and crumbled
- A drizzle of olive oil
- 1 small red onion, chopped
- 1 red bell pepper, chopped
- 1 sweet potato, grated
- 1 green bell pepper, chopped
- 2 garlic cloves, minced
- 1 cup white mushrooms, sliced
- ½ cup quinoa
- 1 cup chicken stock
- 4 eggs, fried
- Salt and black pepper to the taste

Directions:

1. Heat up a pan with the oil over medium-low heat, add the onion, garlic, bell peppers, sweet potato and the mushrooms, toss and sauté for 5 minutes.
2. Add the quinoa, toss and cook for 1 more minute.

3. Add the stock, salt and pepper, stir and cook for 15 minutes.
4. Divide the mix between plates, top each serving with a fried egg, sprinkle some salt, pepper and crumbled bacon and serve for breakfast.

Nutrition:

Calories 304,

Fat 14 g,

Fiber 3.8 g,

Carbs 27.5 g,

Protein 17.8 g

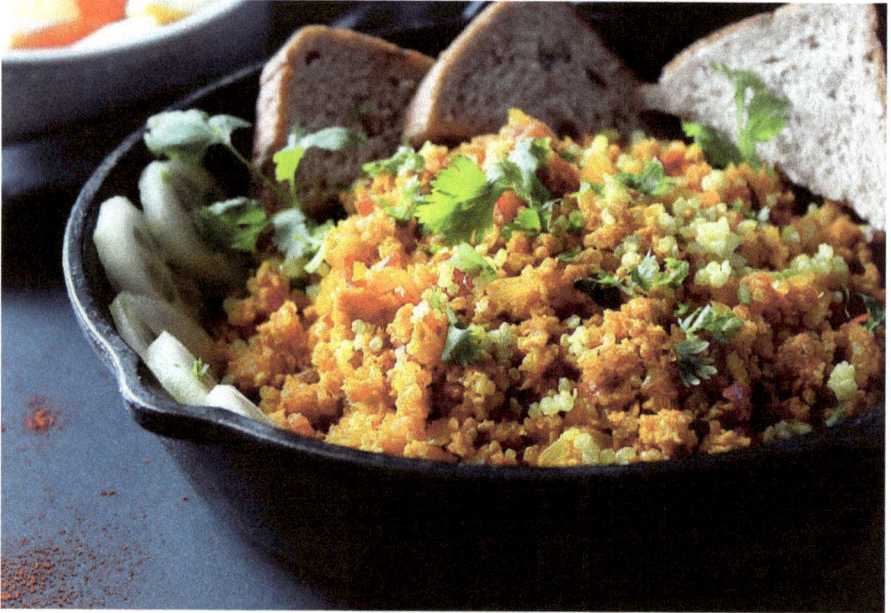

Stuffed Tomatoes

Preparation Time: 10 minutes

Cooking Time: 15 minutes

Servings: 4

Ingredients:

- 2 tbsp. olive oil
- 8 tomatoes, insides scooped
- ¼ cup almond milk
- 8 eggs
- ¼ cup parmesan, grated
- Salt and black pepper to the taste
- 4 tbsp. rosemary, chopped

Directions:

1. Grease a pan with the oil and arrange the tomatoes inside.
2. Crack an egg in each tomato, divide the milk and the rest of the ingredients, introduce the pan in the oven and bake at 375°F for 15 minutes.
3. Serve for breakfast right away.

Nutrition:

Calories 276,

Fat 20.3 g,

Fiber 4.7 g,

Carbs 13.2 g,

Protein 13.7 g

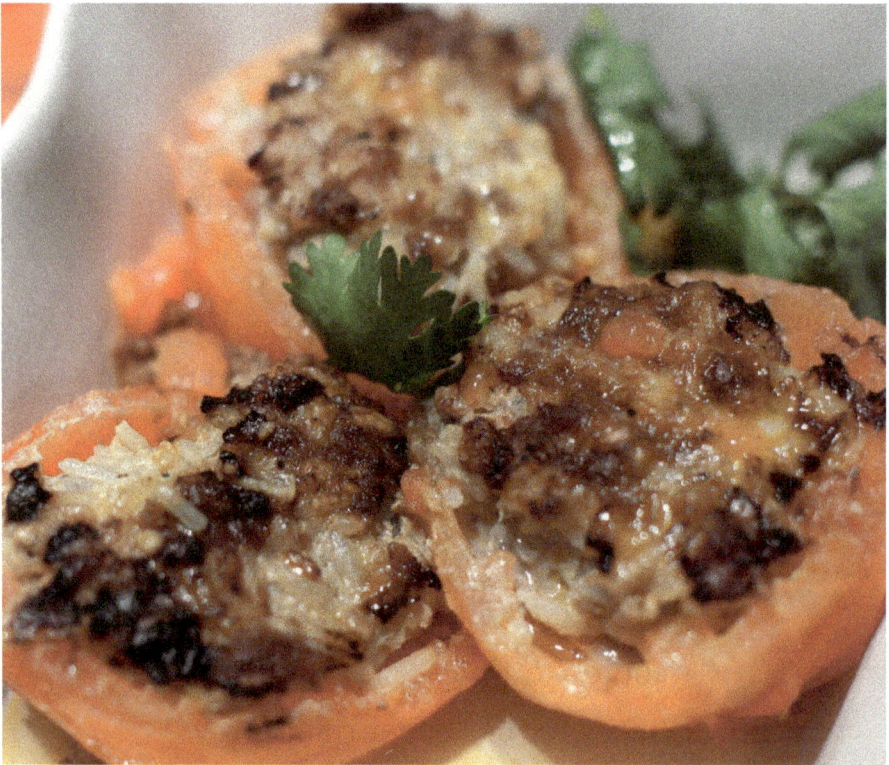

Scrambled Eggs

Preparation Time: 10 minutes

Cooking Time: 10 minutes

Servings: 2

Ingredients:

- 1 yellow bell pepper, chopped
- 8 cherry tomatoes, cubed
- 2 spring onions, chopped
- 1 tbsp. olive oil
- 1 tbsp. capers, drained
- 2 tbsp. black olives, pitted and sliced
- 4 eggs
- A pinch of salt and black pepper
- ¼ tsp. oregano, dried
- 1 tbsp. parsley, chopped

Directions:

1. Heat up a pan with the oil over medium-high heat, add the bell pepper and spring onions and sauté for 3 minutes.
2. Add the tomatoes, capers and the olives and sauté for 2 minutes more.
3. Crack the eggs into the pan, add salt, pepper and the oregano and scramble for 5 minutes more.

4.   Divide the scramble between plates, sprinkle the parsley on top and serve.

Nutrition:

Calories 249,

Fat 17 g,

Fiber 3.2 g,

Carbs 13.3 g,

Protein 13.5 g

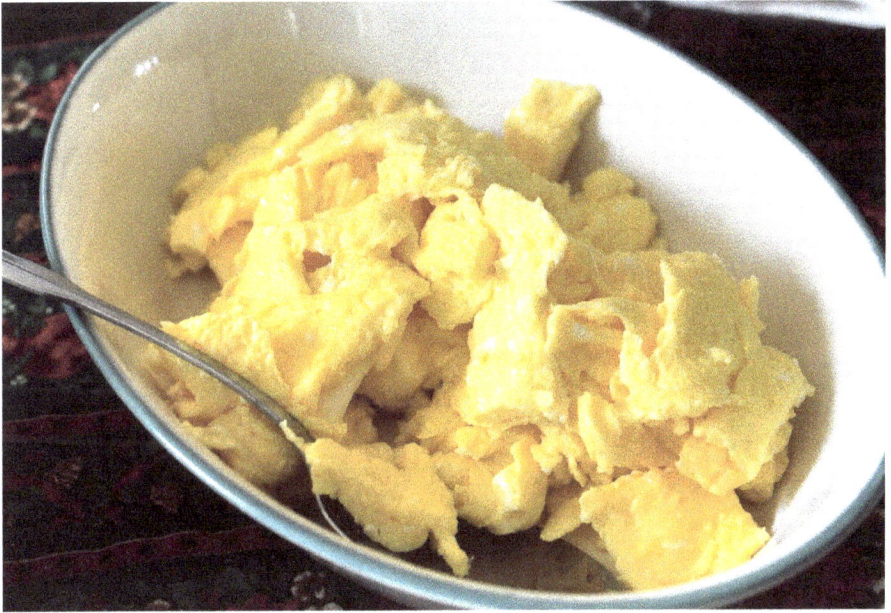

Watermelon "Pizza"

Preparation Time: 10 minutes

Cooking Time: 0 minutes

Servings: 4

Ingredients:

- 1 watermelon slice cut 1-inch thick and then from the center cut into 4 wedges resembling pizza slices
- 6 kalamata olives, pitted and sliced
- 1 oz. feta cheese, crumbled
- ½ tbsp. balsamic vinegar
- 1 tsp. mint, chopped

Directions:

1. Arrange the watermelon "pizza" on a plate, sprinkle the olives and the rest of the ingredients on each slice and serve right away for breakfast.

Nutrition:

Calories 90,

Fat 3 g,

Fiber 1 g,

Carbs 14 g,

Protein 2 g

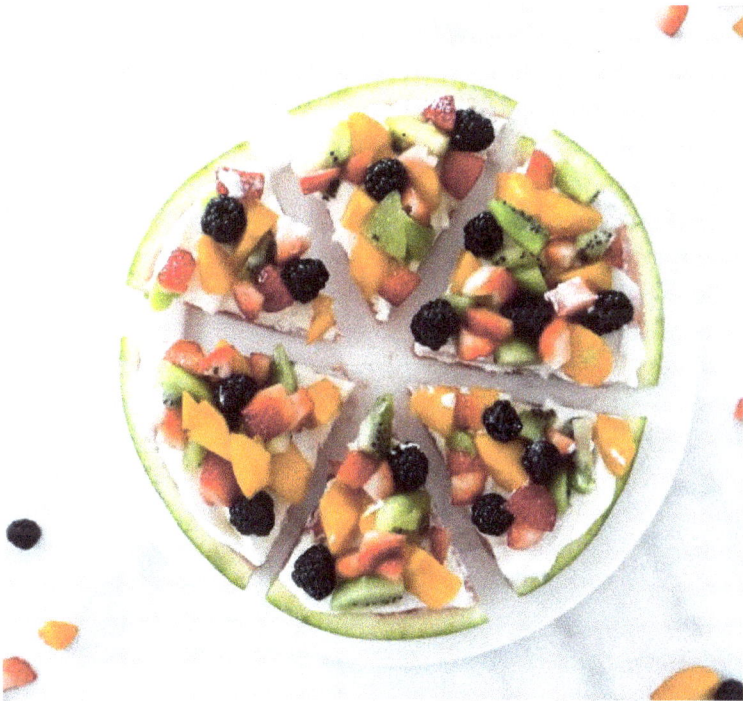

Baked Omelet Mix

Preparation Time: 10 minutes

Cooking Time: 45 minutes

Servings: 12

 Ingredients:

- 12 eggs, whisked
- 8 oz. spinach, chopped
- 2 cups almond milk
- 12 oz. canned artichokes, chopped
- 2 garlic cloves, minced
- 5 oz. feta cheese, crumbled
- 1 tbsp. dill, chopped
- 1 tsp. oregano, dried
- 1 tsp. lemon pepper
- A pinch of salt
- 4 tsp. olive oil

Directions:

1. Heat up a pan with the oil over medium-high heat, add the garlic and the spinach and sauté for 3 minutes.
2. In a baking dish, combine the eggs with the artichokes and the rest of the ingredients.

3.   Add the spinach mix as well, toss a bit, bake the mix at 375°F for 40 minutes, divide between plates and serve for breakfast.

Nutrition:

Calories 186,

Fat 13 g,

Fiber 1 g,

Carbs 5 g,

Protein 10 g

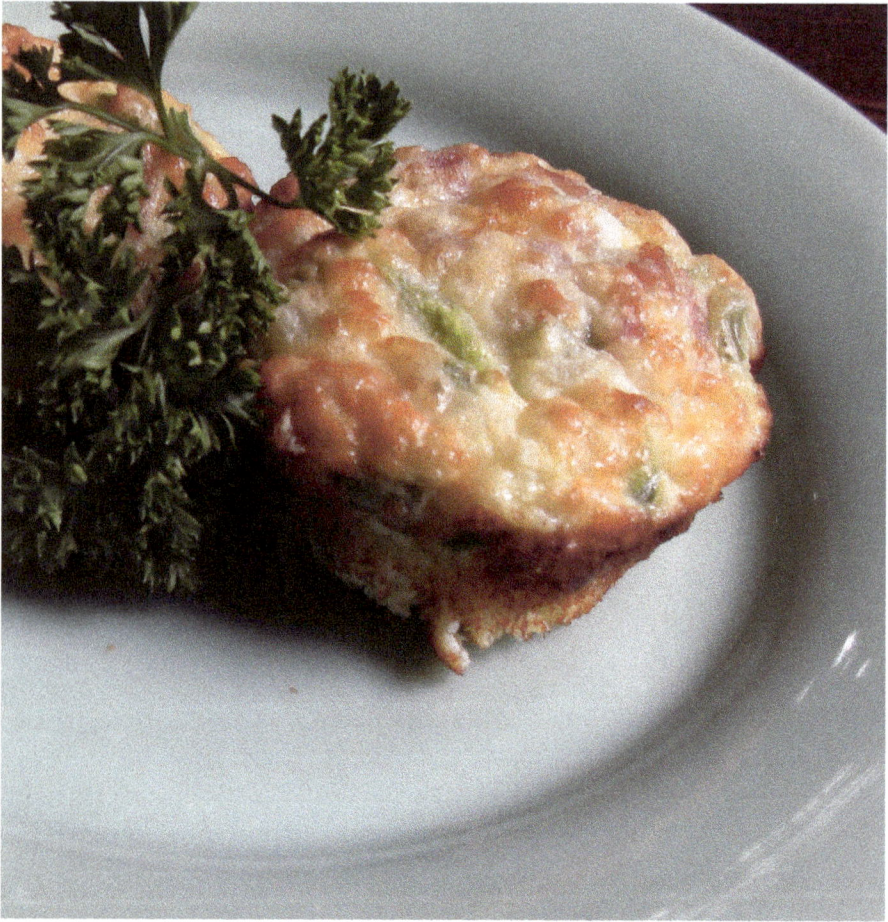

Anti-Inflammatory Blueberry Smoothie

Preparation Time: 5 minutes

Cooking Time: 5 minutes

Servings: 1

Ingredients:

- Almond milk (1 cup)
- Frozen banana (1)
- Frozen blueberries (2/3-1 cup)
- Leafy greens/spinach (2 handfuls)
- Almond butter (1 tbsp.)
- Cinnamon (.25 tsp.)
- Cayenne pepper (.125-.25 tsp.)
- Optional: Maca powder (1 tsp.)

Directions:

1. Combine each of the fixings using a high-powered blender.

2. Mix thoroughly until creamy and serve in a chilled glass.

Nutrition:

Calories: 340

Protein: 9 g

Fat: 13 g

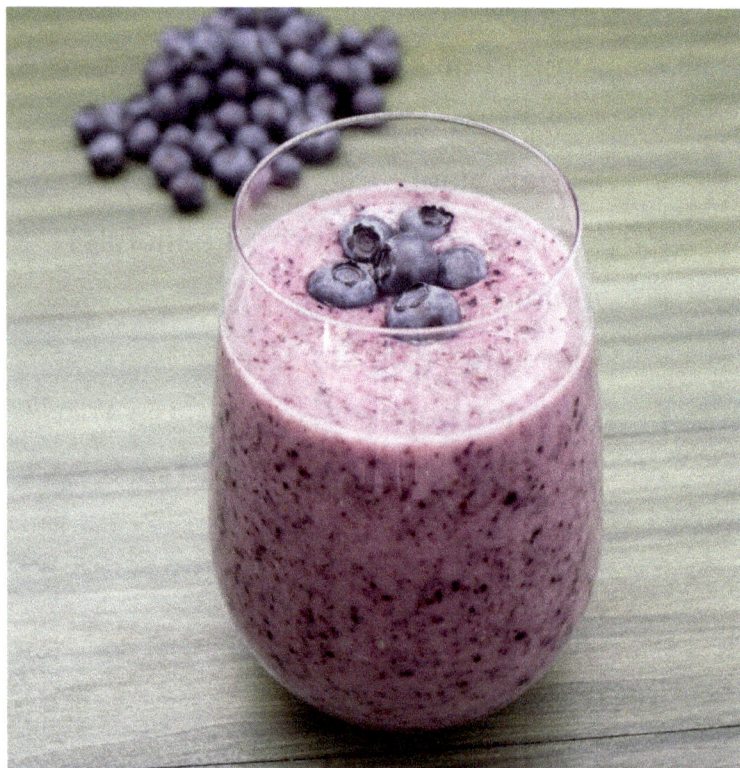

Cherry - Pomegranate Smoothie Bow - Gluten-Free & Vegetarian

Preparation Time: 5 minutes

Cooking Time: 5 minutes

Servings: 4

Ingredients:

- Frozen dark sweet cherries (16 oz. bag)
- 2% Plain Greek yogurt (1.5 cups)
- Pomegranate juice (.75 cup)
- 2% milk (.33 cup (+) more as needed)
- Ground cinnamon (.75 tsp.)
- Vanilla extract (1 tsp.)
- Fresh pomegranate seeds (.5 cup)
- Chopped pistachios (.5 cup)
- Ice cubes (6)

Directions:

1. Chop the pistachios or purchase (arils) found in the produce section of the market. If you are using the whole fruit, remove the seeds underwater in a container so they will float to the top.

2.   Add the fixings into a blender (ice, milk, cinnamon, vanilla, juice, yogurt, and cherries).
3.   Pulse until it's creamy smooth. Use a little extra milk to thin the texture to get it to the desired consistency.
4.   Pour the prepared smoothie into for dishes and top with two tbsp. of the chopped pistachios and two tbsp. of the seeds. Serve it immediately.

Nutrition:

Calories: 212

Protein: 4 g

Fat: 7 g

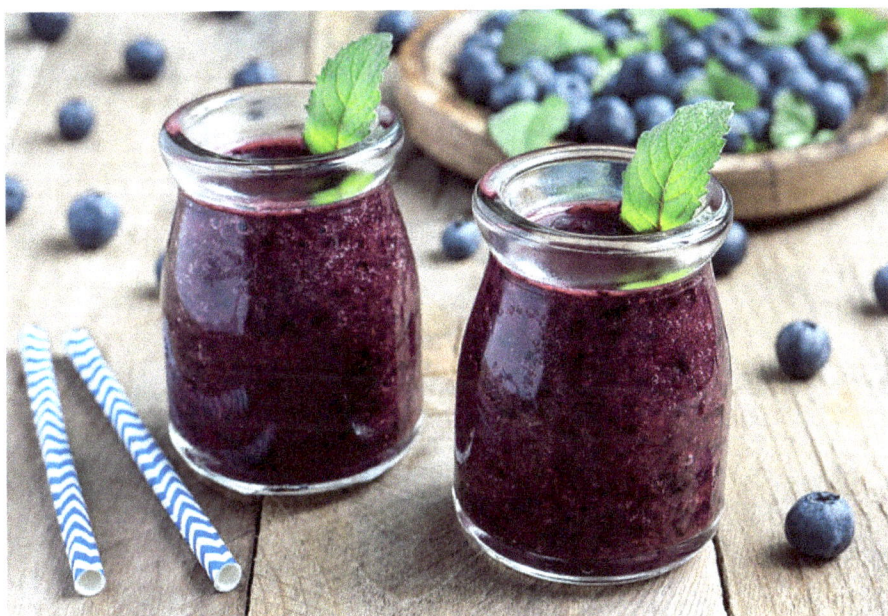

Breakfast Banana Green Smoothie

Preparation Time: 5 minutes

Cooking Time: 5 minutes

Servings: 1

Ingredients:

- 2 cups baby spinach leaves, or to taste
- 1 banana
- 1 carrot, peeled and cut into large chunks
- ¾ cup plain Fat-free Greek yogurt, or to taste
- ¾ cup ice
- 2 tbsp. honey

Directions:

1. Put spinach, banana, carrot, yogurt, ice, and honey in a blender; blend until smooth.
2. Enjoy!

Nutrition:

Calories: 212

Protein: 4 g

Fat: 7 g

Strawberry Oatmeal Breakfast Smoothie

Preparation Time: 5 minutes

Cooking Time: 5 minutes

Servings: 2

Ingredients:

- 1 cup soy milk
- ½ cup rolled oats
- 1 banana, broken into chunks
- 14 frozen strawberries
- ½ tsp. vanilla extract
- 1 ½ tsp. white sugar

Directions:

1. In a blender, combine soy milk, oats, banana and strawberries. Add vanilla and sugar if desired. Blend until smooth.
2. Pour into glasses and serve.

Nutrition:

Calories: 232

Protein: 4 g

Fat: 5 g

Kale and Banana Smoothie

Preparation Time: 5 minutes

Cooking Time: 5 minutes

Servings: 1

Ingredients:

- 1 banana
- 2 cups chopped kale
- ½ cup light unsweetened soy milk
- 1 tbsp. flax seeds
- 1 tsp. maple syrup

Directions:

1. Place the banana, kale, soy milk, flax seeds, and maple syrup into a blender. Cover, and puree until smooth. Serve over ice.

Nutrition:

Calories: 221

Protein: 3 g

Fat: 7 g

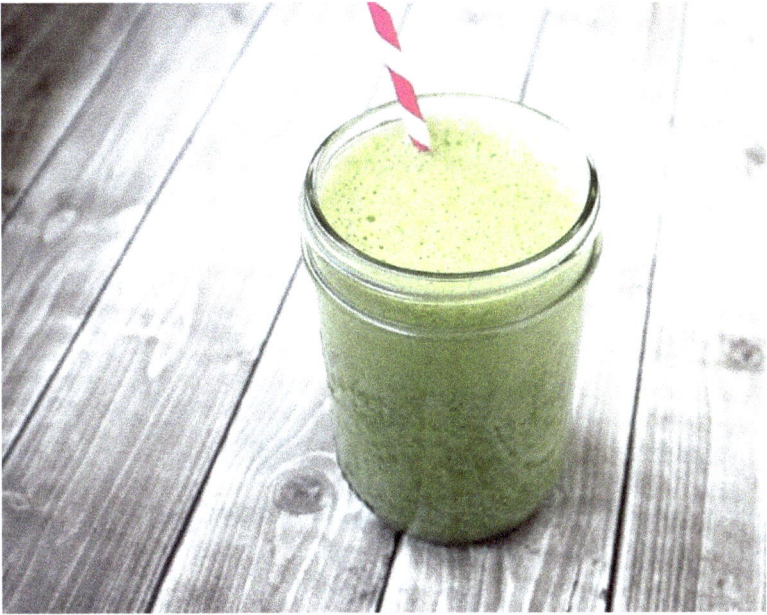

Summer Stone Fruit Smoothie

Preparation Time: 5 minutes

Cooking Time: 0 minutes

Servings: 2

Ingredients:

- ½ cup Greek yogurt
- 1 plum, pit removed, flesh roughly chopped
- 1 peach, pit removed, flesh roughly chopped
- 1 nectarine, pit removed, flesh roughly chopped
- ½ cup blueberries, fresh or frozen

Directions:

1. Combine all ingredients in blender and blend until smooth.
2. Enjoy!

Nutrition:

Calories: 212

Protein: 4 g

Fat: 7 g

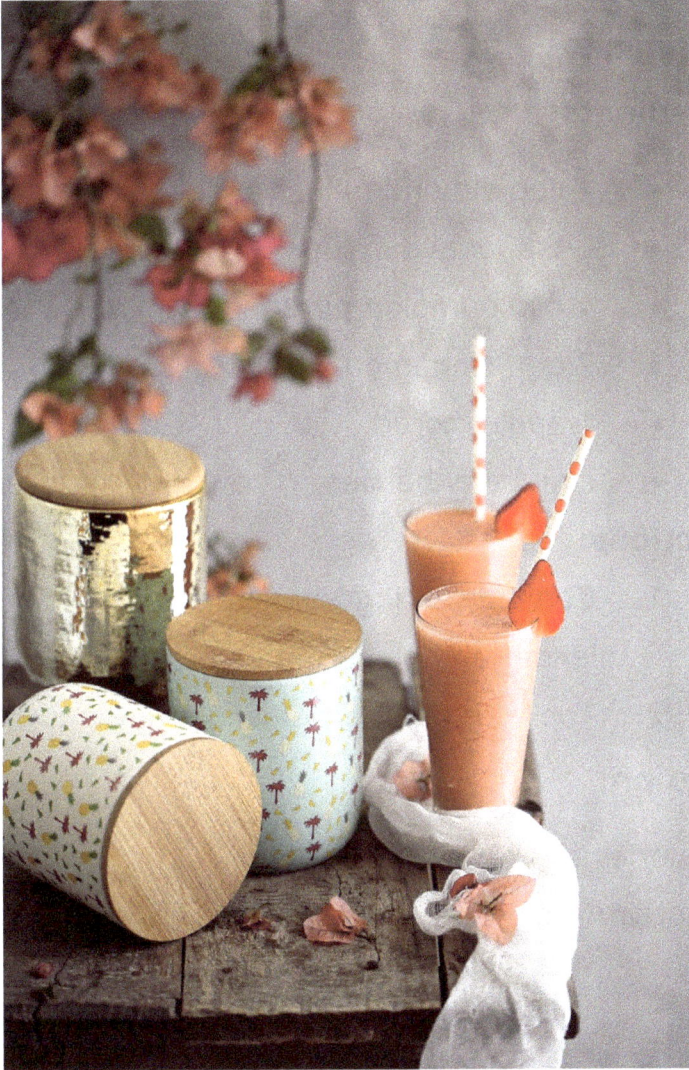

Pumpkin Pie Fall Smoothie

Preparation Time: 5 minutes

Cooking Time: 0 minutes

Servings: 3

Ingredients:

- 1 cup almond milk
- 1 tsp. agave syrup
- 1 cup pumpkin puree
- 2 tsp. cinnamon
- 1 apple, cored
- Dried cranberries

Directions:

1. Combine all ingredients except cranberries in blender and blend until smooth.
2. Top with cranberries and enjoy.

Nutrition:

Calories: 231

Protein: 4 g

Fat: 6 g

Green Tart Smoothie

Preparation Time: 5 minutes

Cooking Time: 5 minutes

Servings: 1

Ingredients:

- 2 cups fresh kale
- 1 cup water
- 2 large stalks of celery, chopped
- ½ cucumber, chopped
- 1/3 grapefruit
- 1 cup frozen pineapple

Directions:

1. Blend kale and water until smooth.
2. Add remaining ingredients, and blend until smooth.
3. Enjoy!

Nutrition:

Calories: 214

Protein: 4 g

Fat: 7 g

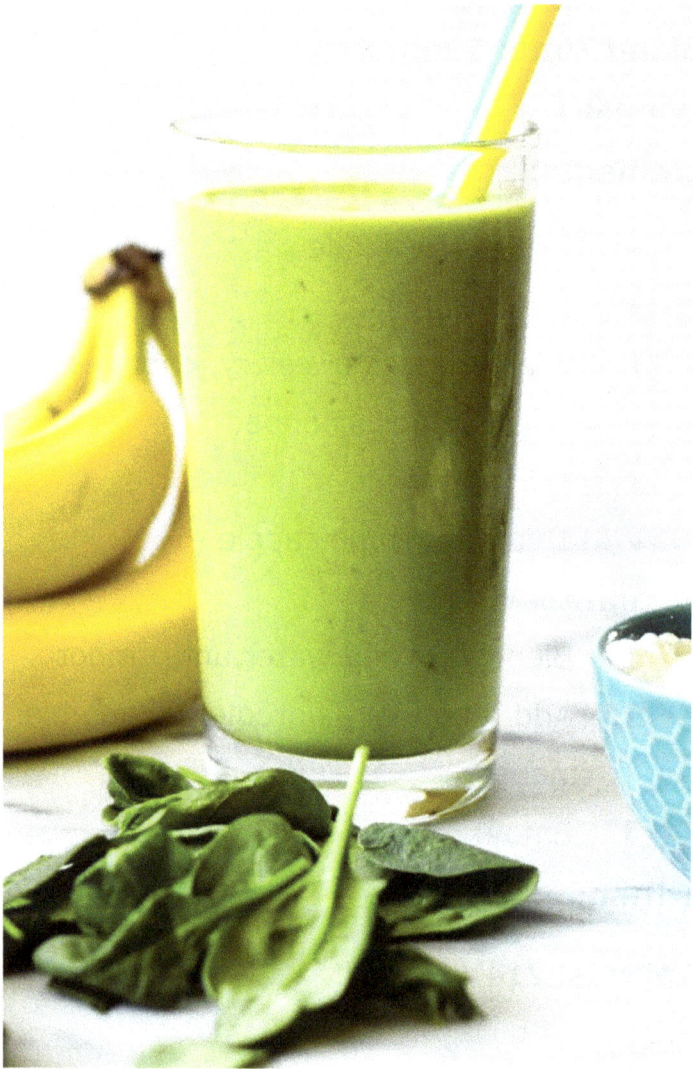

Coconut Milk Smoothie

Preparation Time: 10 minutes

Cooking Time: 0 minutes

Servings: 1

Ingredients:

- 1 1/2 cups coconut milk
- 1 frozen banana
- 2 cups raw baby spinach

Directions:

1. Add everything to a food processor.
2. Blend the ingredients well until smooth.
3. Refrigerate until chilled enough.
4. Serve with your favorite garnish

Nutrition:

Calories: 212

Protein: 4 g

Fat: 7 g

Creamy Strawberry Smoothie

Preparation Time: 10 minutes

Cooking Time: 0 minutes

Servings: 1

Ingredients:

- 1 banana
- 1/2 cup frozen strawberries
- 1/2 cup frozen mango
- 1/2 cup Greek yogurt
- 1/4 cup coconut milk
- 1/4 tsp. turmeric
- 1/4 tsp. ginger
- 1 tbsp. honey

Directions:

1. Add everything to a food processor.
2. Blend the ingredients well until smooth.
3. Refrigerate until chilled enough.
4. Serve with your favorite garnish

Nutrition:

Calories: 237

Protein: 4 g

Fat: 3 g

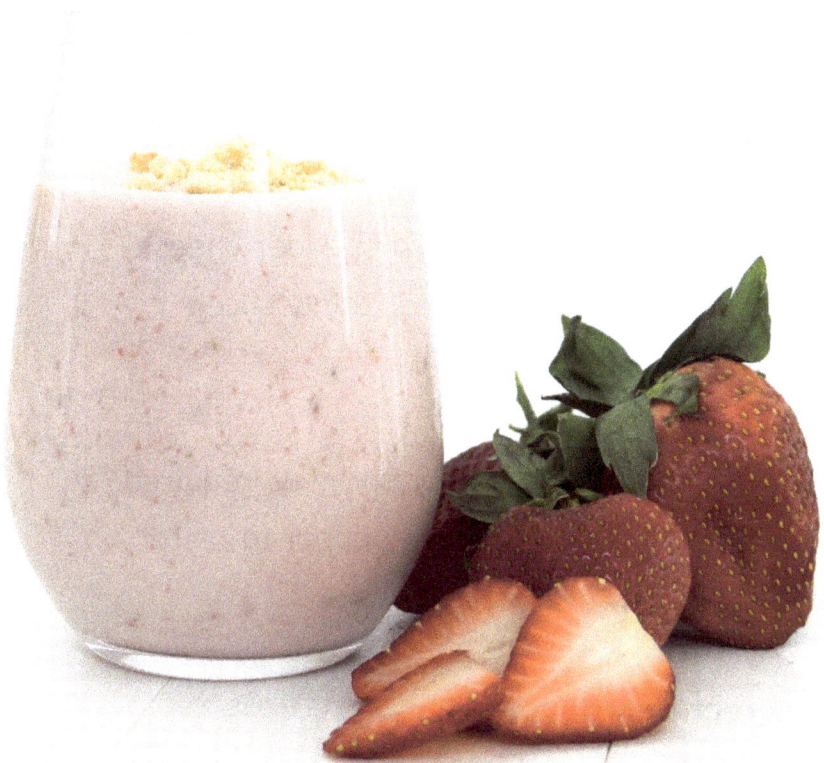

Cheddar Potato Crisps

Preparation Time: 10 minutes

Cooking Time: 0 minutes

Servings: 4

Ingredients:

- 1 cup Greek yogurt (unsweetened)
- 1/2 cup grated cheddar cheese
- 6 red potatoes, thinly sliced
- 1/2 cup chives
- 3 slices ham
- Cooking oil or spray as required
- Salt and black pepper to taste

Directions:

1. Take the potatoes; sprinkle with salt and black pepper.
2. Cover and place in the refrigerator for 30 minutes.
3. Heat a grill at medium temperature setting.

4. Spray the potato slices with cooking oil, place over a baking sheet and grill for about 2 minutes.

5. Flip and grill for 2 more minutes. Add the ham slices to the baking sheet and grill for one minute.

6. Add the potato and ham in a serving bowl. Top with the chives, yogurt and grated cheese as desired.

Nutrition: Calories – 494 | Fat – 18g | Carbs – 46g | Fiber – 9g | Protein – 24g

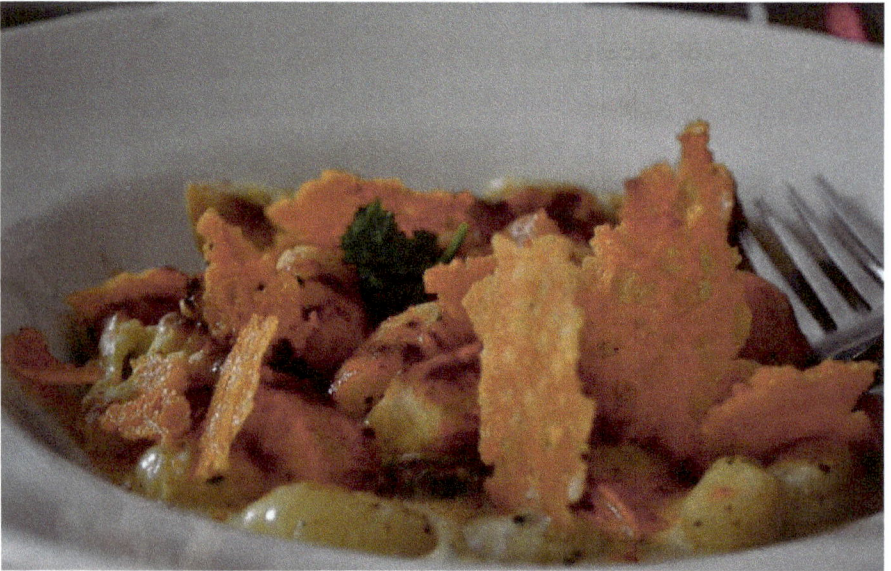

Stuffed Sweet Potato

Preparation Time: 10 minutes

Cooking Time: 40 minutes

Servings: 8

Ingredients:

- 8 sweet potatoes, pierced with a fork
- 14 oz. canned chickpeas, drained and rinsed
- 1 small red bell pepper, chopped
- 1 tbsp. lemon zest, grated
- 2 tbsp. lemon juice
- 3 tbsp. olive oil
- 1 tsp. garlic, minced
- 1 tbsp. oregano, chopped
- 2 tbsp. parsley, chopped
- A pinch of salt and black pepper
- 1 avocado, peeled, pitted and mashed
- ¼ cup water
- ¼ cup tahini paste

Directions:

1. Arrange the potatoes on a baking sheet lined with parchment paper, bake them at 400°F for 40 minutes, cool them down and cut a slit down the middle in each.

2.   In a bowl, combine the chickpeas with the bell pepper, lemon zest, half of the lemon juice, half of the oil, half of the garlic, oregano, half of the parsley, salt and pepper, toss and stuff the potatoes with this mix.

3.   In another bowl, mix the avocado with the water, tahini, the rest of the lemon juice, oil, garlic and parsley, whisk well and spread over the potatoes.

4.   Serve cold for breakfast.

Nutrition:

Calories 308,

Fat 2 g,

Fiber 8 g,

Carbs 38 g,

Protein 7 g

Rosemary Bulgur Appetizer

Preparation Time: 25 minutes

Cooking Time: 0 minutes

Servings: 6

Ingredients:

- ½ cup couscous
- 2 tbsp. olive oil
- 1 ¾ cup onions, chopped
- 2 cups vegetable broth
- 1 cup bulgur
- 1 tbsp. chives, chopped
- 1 tbsp. parsley, chopped
- ¼ tsp. rosemary, chopped

Directions:

1. Over medium stove flame; heat the oil in a skillet or saucepan (preferably medium size).
2. Sauté the onions until softened and translucent, stir in between.

3. Add the bulgur and 1 ½ cups vegetable broth; simmer the mixture until the bulgur is tender.
4. Remove it from the heat and fluff with a fork.
5. In another skillet or saucepan, heat the remaining vegetable broth and simmer. Add the oil and couscous. Stir and cook this until your couscous is tender. Fluff it with a fork.
6. In a mixing bowl, combine the bulgur and couscous. Add the rosemary, chives and parsley on top. Season it with black pepper and salt.
7. Serve as an appetizer or light meal.

Nutrition: Calories – 182 |Fat – 6g|Carbs – 28g|Fiber – 4g|Protein – 8g

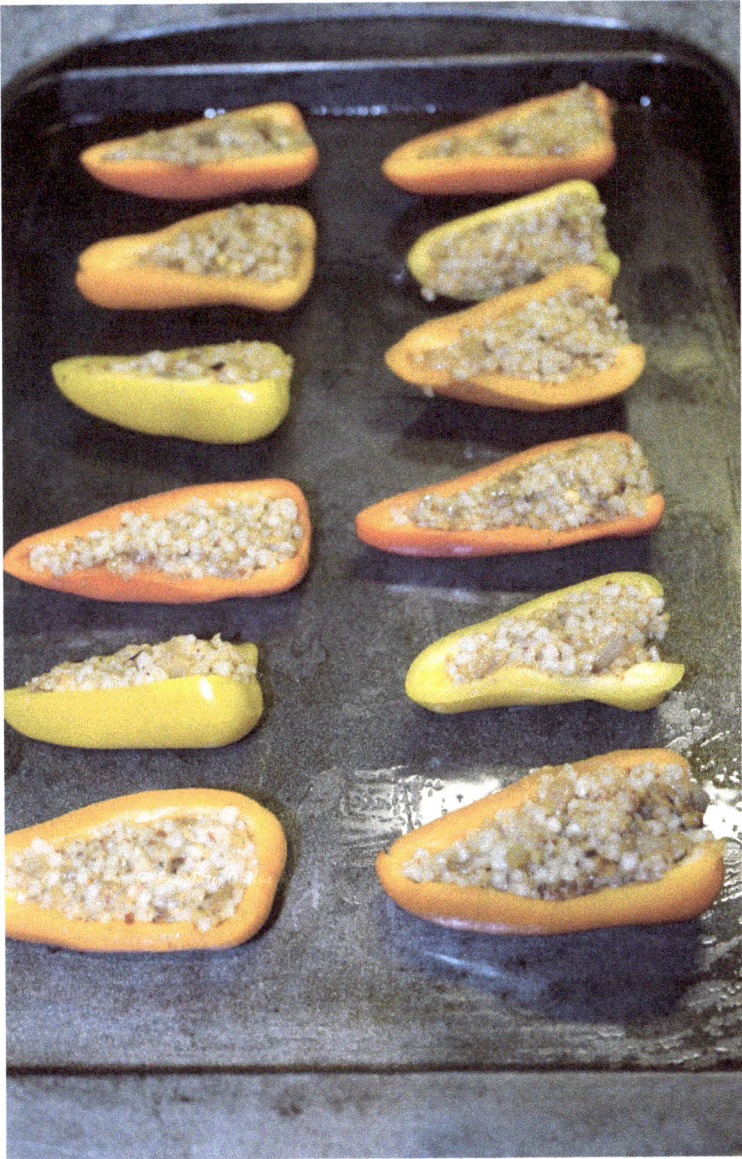

Cauliflower Fritters

Preparation Time: 10 minutes

Cooking Time: 50 minutes

Servings: 4

Ingredients:

- 30 oz. canned chickpeas, drained and rinsed
- 2 and ½ tbsp. olive oil
- 1 small yellow onion, chopped
- 2 cups cauliflower florets chopped
- 2 tbsp. garlic, minced
- A pinch of salt and black pepper

Directions:

1. Spread half of the chickpeas on a baking sheet lined with parchment pepper, add 1 tbsp. oil, season with salt and pepper, toss and bake at 400°F for 30 minutes.
2. Transfer the chickpeas to a food processor, pulse well and put the mix into a bowl.
3. Heat up a pan with the ½ tbsp. oil over medium-high heat, add the garlic and the onion and sauté for 3 minutes.
4. Add the cauliflower, cook for 6 minutes more, transfer this to a blender, add the rest of the chickpeas, pulse, pour over the crispy

chickpeas mix from the bowl, stir and shape medium fritters out of this mix.

5. Heat up a pan with the rest of the oil over medium-high heat, add the fritters, cook them for 3 minutes on each side and serve for breakfast.

Nutrition:

Calories 333,

Fat 12.6 g,

Fiber 12.8 g,

Carbs 44.7 g,

Protein 13.6 g

Mediterranean Chickpea Snack

Preparation Time: 30 minutes

Cooking Time: 0 minutes

Servings: 2

Ingredients:

- ½ tsp. garlic powder
- 1 can (10 oz.) chickpeas, rinsed and drained
- ½ tsp. dried basil
- 1 tsp. extra-virgin olive oil
- ¼ tsp. sea salt
- 1 tsp. Nutritional Yeast
- ¼ tsp. red pepper flakes

Directions:

1. Preheat the oven to 450°F. Line a baking pan with a parchment paper. Grease it with some refined coconut oil or avocado oil (You can also use cooking spray)

2. Combine the chickpeas, seasonings, and oil in a mixing bowl.

3. Arrange the chickpeas in the pan. Roast the chickpeas for about 10 minutes. Toss and keep roasting for 10 more minutes.

4. Serve warm.

Nutrition: Calories – 321|Fat – 8g|Carbs – 42g|Fiber – 12g|Protein – 22g

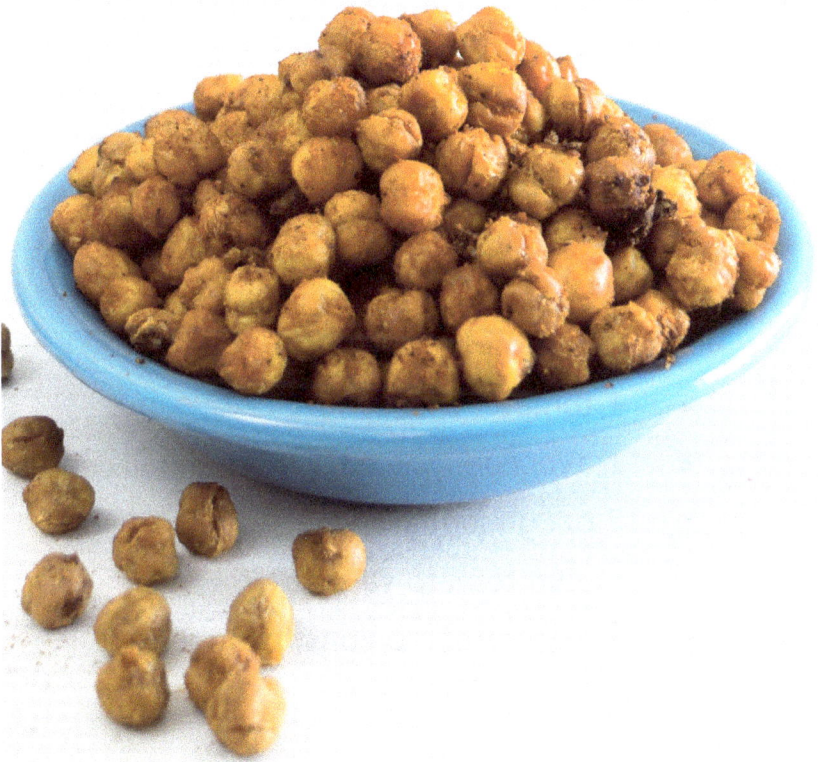

Avocado Chickpea Pizza

Preparation Time: 20 minutes

Cooking Time: 20 minutes

Servings: 2

Ingredients:

- 1 and ¼ cups chickpea flour
- A pinch of salt and black pepper
- 1 and ¼ cups water
- 2 tbsp. olive oil
- 1 tsp. onion powder
- 1 tsp. garlic, minced
- 1 tomato, sliced
- 1 avocado, peeled, pitted and sliced
- 2 oz. gouda, sliced
- ¼ cup tomato sauce
- 2 tbsp. green onions, chopped

Directions:

1. In a bowl, mix the chickpea flour with salt, pepper, water, the oil, onion powder and the garlic, stir well until you obtain a dough,

knead a bit, put in a bowl, cover and leave aside for 20 minutes.

2. Transfer the dough to a working surface, shape a bit circle, transfer it to a baking sheet lined with parchment paper and bake at 425°F for 10 minutes.

3. Spread the tomato sauce over the pizza, also spread the rest of the ingredients and bake at 400°F for 10 minutes more.

4. Cut and serve for breakfast.

Nutrition:

Calories 416,

Fat 24.5 g,

Fiber 9.6 g,

Carbs 36.6 g,

Protein 15.4 g

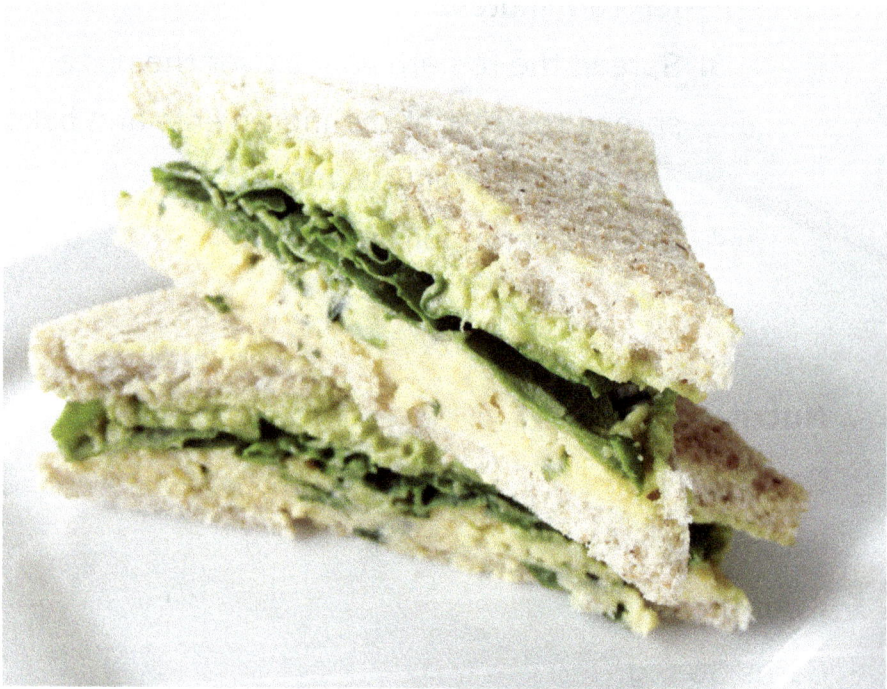

Pita Wedges with Almond Bean Dip

Preparation Time: 10 minutes

Cooking Time: 5 minutes

Servings: 5

Ingredients:

- 8 oz. beet, cubed
- 5 garlic cloves, peeled
- ¼ cup almond, slivered
- 15 ½ oz. garbanzo beans
- ¾ cup extra-virgin olive oil
- 1 ½ tbsp. red wine vinegar
- Whole-wheat pita wedges to serve

Directions:

1. In a saucepan or deep skillet, boil the beet in sufficient quantity of water until it is tender. Drain, peel, cut in cubes and blend in a food processor.
2. Add the garbanzo beans, almonds, oil, and garlic and blend everything well until smooth. Add the red wine and blend for one more minute.
3. Season with black pepper and salt. Chill in the refrigerator. Serve with pita wedges.

Nutrition: Calories – 356|Fat – 21g|Carbs – 23g|Fiber – 6g|Protein – 6g

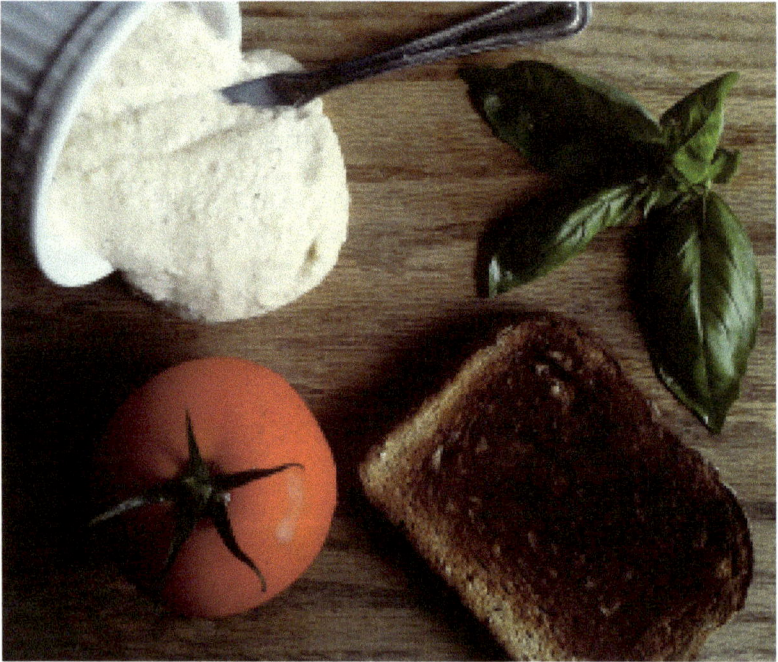

Ginger Antipasti

Preparation Time: 10 minutes

Cooking Time: 0 minutes

Servings: 6

Ingredients:

- 1 tsp. ginger powder
- 1 cup fresh parsley, chopped
- 1 tbsp. apple cider vinegar
- 3 tbsp. avocado oil
- 2 oz celery stalk, chopped

Directions:

1. Mix all ingredients in the bowl and leave for 5 minutes in the fridge.

Nutrition: Calories 16g, Protein 0.5g, Carbs 1.5g, Fat 1g

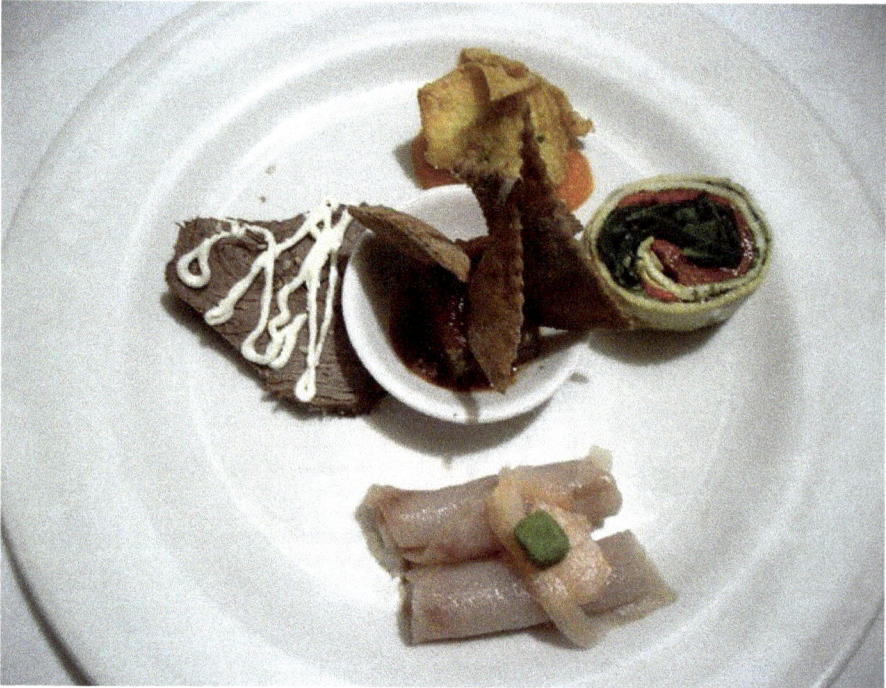

Mediterranean Chickpea Spread

Preparation Time: 8 minutes

Cooking Time: 5 minutes

Servings: 2

Ingredients:

- 2 cups chickpeas (canned or pre-soaked and cooked)
- 2 tbsp. lemon juice
- 1/2 tsp. cumin
- 2 cloves garlic, minced
- 4 tsp. olive oil
- Salt to taste
- Ground cinnamon (optional)

Directions:

1. In a mixing bowl, add the chickpeas; mash thoroughly using a fork (you can also use a blender).
2. Add the olive oil, garlic and lemon juice. Combine well; top with some cinnamon.
3. Serve with vegetable sticks, whole-wheat crackers, or whole-wheat pita wedges.

Nutrition: Calories – 412|Fat – 11g|Carbs – 34g|Fiber – 14g|Protein – 20g

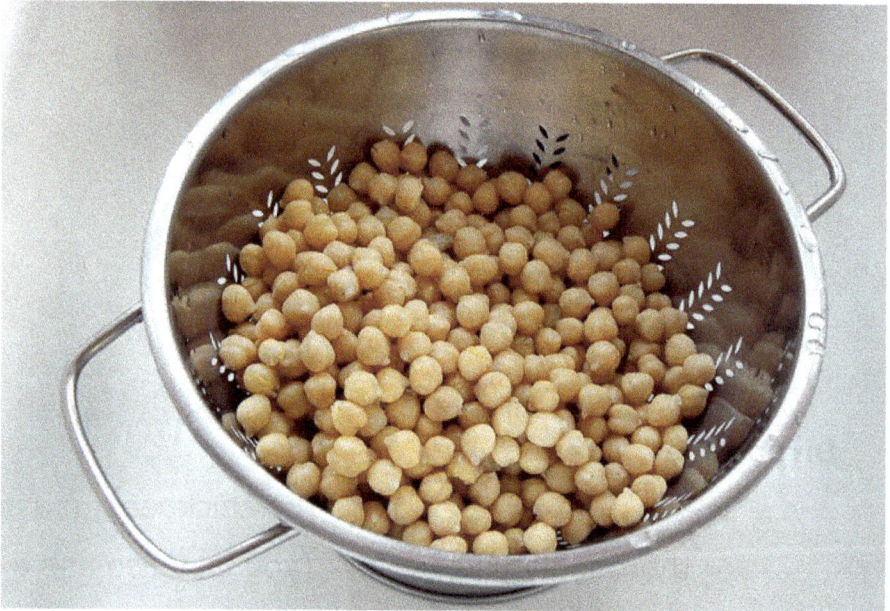

Rosemary Beets

Preparation Time: 10 minutes

Cooking Time: 4 minutes

Servings: 6

Ingredients:

- 1-lb. beets, sliced, peeled
- 2 tbsp. lemon juice
- 1 tsp. dried rosemary
- ¼ tsp. garlic powder
- 1 tbsp. olive oil

Directions:

1. Sprinkle the beets with lemon juice, rosemary, garlic powder, and olive oil.
2. Then preheat the grill to 400°F.
3. Place the sliced beet in the grill and cook it for 2 minutes per side.

Nutrition: 56 Calories, 1.3g Protein, 7.9g Carbs, 2.5g Fat, 1.6g Fiber

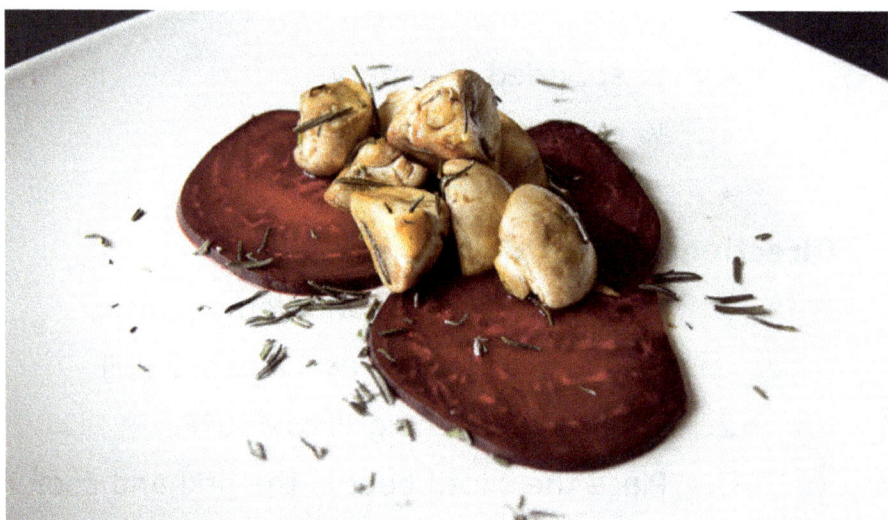

Scallions Dip

Preparation Time: 5 minutes

Cooking Time: 15 minutes

Servings: 4

Ingredients:

- 1 cup spinach, chopped
- 2 oz scallions, chopped
- ¼ cup plain yogurt
- ¼ tsp. chili powder
- 1 tsp. olive oil

Directions:

1. Melt the olive oil in the saucepan.
2. Add spinach and scallions.
3. Saute the greens for 10 minutes.
4. Then add chili powder and plain yogurt. Stir well and cook it for 5 minutes more.
5. Then blend the mixture with the help of the immersion blender.

Nutrition: 27 Calories, 1.4g Protein, 2.5g Carbs, 1.4g Fat, 0.6g Fiber

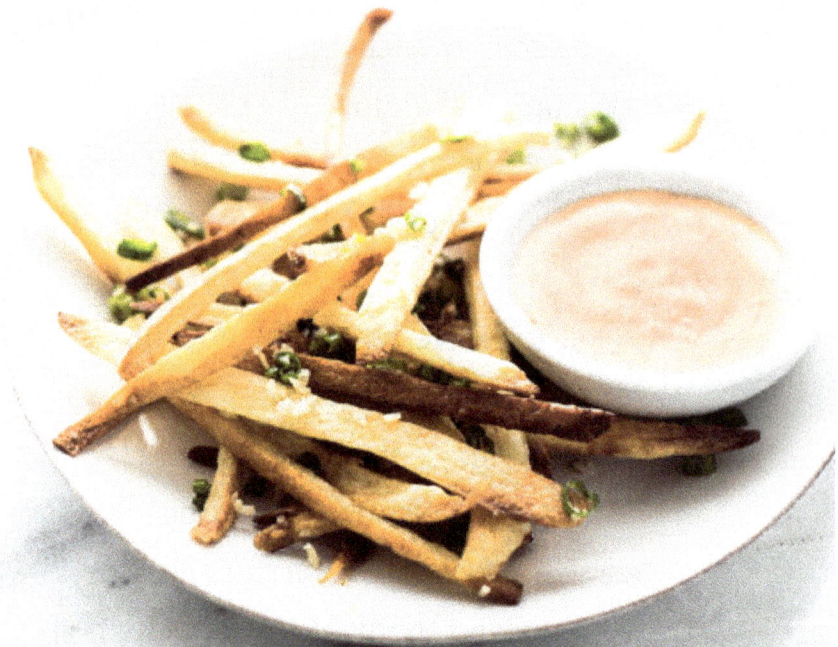

www.ingramcontent.com/pod-product-compliance
Lightning Source LLC
Chambersburg PA
CBHW050754030426
42336CB00012B/1809